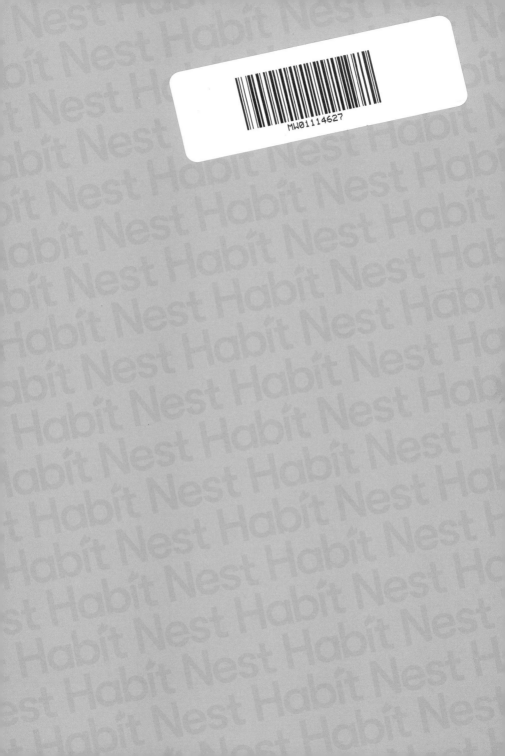

ISBN: 9781950045266   Transformation Journal: **First Edition**

Volume 1

Home Organization Transformation Journal

Finally become clutter-free.

Habit Nest

Small Steps, Finally person you

Big Changes.
become the
want to be.

Better habits made simple.

Journey Overview

Let's Get
Started

You're likely here because you're motivated and ready for change.

Maybe you've tried to declutter and organize your home in the past and saw some progress, but life got in the way. Or perhaps amidst the chaos of your busy routine, you couldn't figure out how to realistically make your home work for you.

Just as millions of others have made lasting changes using the systems found in this journal, so can you.

This whole journey is designed around one simple idea: Show up on the good days and the bad, just as you have today.

Why? Because becoming clutter-free is inevitable when you're someone who consistently shows up.

This Habit-Building System Will Help You:

Save valuable time

Accelerate your learning curve.
Our team conducted 1,000+
hours of research so you
don't have to.

Make habit building feel simple and easy

Know exactly what to do, when.
See real results without
the struggle.

Fit your new routine into your existing lifestyle

Designed to work for everybody,
no matter what your life looks like.

Stay engaged and see tangible growth

Uncover a treasure trove of
content & resources designed
to be directly actionable.

As you start this journey,
make one simple commitment to yourself:

Open This
Journal

Each day you commit to completing your home organization journey, simply focus on taking this one small step.

While this single action won't literally make your home clutter-free and organized, it has a powerful purpose: to make it easy to show up and take the next steps needed to get you there.

In time, this single action will grow into real results.

Making Consistency Easy

To reliably open this journal each day, you'll have to know where to find it.

Keep it in a prominent and visible place, ideally somewhere related to the next steps of your journey, such as a prominent place in the room you are organizing.

Where will you keep this journal?

....

Next, let's establish a clear and specific signal, or habit cue, for when you will open your journal and continue your home organization journey. There are multiple types of habit cues you can use for this:

- **Time:** At a specific time each day (e.g. an alarm that goes off at a set time)
- **Location:** When you arrive at a specific place (e.g. when you walk into your living room)
- **Habit Stack:** Follow up an existing daily behavior (e.g. brushing your teeth or making morning coffee)

Example of a bad cue: *Each morning, I will open my journal.*

Example of a good cue: *After I walk out of my bathroom in the morning, I will walk to my living room and open my journal.*

Detail your habit cue below. *Remember to make it specific.*

Bookmark this section

Flip back here next time you're struggling to stay consistent.

Define Your Why

The foundation of a lasting home organization journey is knowing what drives you.

Whether it's comfort, functionality, or aesthetics, your 'Why' becomes your guiding compass, especially during more challenging times.

What's the main feeling or desire pushing you on your home organization journey?

Things to consider: how does being clutter-free tie into your overall life goals, values, specific life events or experiences, and any deeper motivations.

The Secret to Behavior Change

The secret to profound and lasting change is not about checking off a to-do each day or reaching a set goal.

It's about evolving your identity.

Embracing identity-based habits means changing from the inside out. When your beliefs about yourself change, your behaviors follow.

So how exactly do you evolve your identity? Simple: You take actions that align with who you want to become.

Each small step you take builds trust with yourself that you are who you aspire to be.

Perfection isn't the goal; consistency is.

Over time, your small actions will solidify into sustainable habits that will reinforce your new identity.

Take a moment to reflect on the person you aspire to be.

Consider that person's core beliefs, their relationship with clutter, organization and home, and their motivations to show up consistently.

Share the vision of who you're becoming with the world using #HabitNest

Planning Ahead

So far you've established **what** you're doing to kick off this habit, **when** you will do so, **why** you're doing this, and **who** you want to become from the process.

Now, we're going to iron out **how** you will fit this routine into your life.

Rather than relying on willpower or your (often unreliable) future self to make all the right decisions, let's instead create a clear plan for you to follow.

With this plan, you sidestep future guesswork, prepare to overcome typical hurdles, and solidify your path to consistency.

Note that you'll have many chances to fine-tune this plan throughout your journey: section reflections will offer more immediate adjustments, while specific milestones will prompt deeper reassessments.

Things to Consider:

1. What days of the week will you do this habit?

2. How will you manage weekends?

3. How do you plan to continue your home organization journey around special occasions, such as holidays or family gatherings?

4. How will you address unexpected interruptions like children, pets, or dependents?

5. How will you handle days when you're not feeling well?

6. How will you adapt your plan if your schedule changes?

7. Will your cue to open this journal ever not be applicable? If so, what will your plan be?

8. Are there any commitments you may need to reprioritize or change?

Create your plan for how this home organization journey will fit into your life.

Use the "Things To Consider" questions on the previous page to establish your own solid habit foundation, personalized to match your lifestyle.

I commit
becoming

**Get Held
Accountable**

to
clutter-free.

I will prove this is who I am by taking small actions to back it up.

I will see this journey through.

_____   _____

SIGNED   DATE

Get The
Most Out of
Your Journal

As you flip through the journal, you'll spot QR codes linking you to additional content and tools tailored specifically for that page.

Habit Nest

Scan here to digitally
enable your habit journey.

How This Journal Works

This journal organizes your home transformation into nine straightforward milestones. The journey targets eight key home areas, ending with a plan to maintain your home.

Your Focus Areas:

Living Room, Kitchen, Bedrooms, Clothing + Accessories, Bathroom, Misc. Indoors, Garage, Everything Outdoors, and Maintenance Plan.

Before beginning each area, you'll set your goals and intentions for that space.

Each main area is broken down into bite-sized categories for focused attention—like separating the Kitchen into 'Countertops' and 'Fridge & Freezer.'

This approach taps into the Goal Gradient Hypothesis, suggesting that smaller, closer goals boost your motivation, making the decluttering journey feel more achievable and rewarding.

Each room contains a discard checklist, followed by an organization guide:

☐ Discard

Simplify your entryway to enhance its welcoming vibe. Remove items that don't belong or no longer serve a purpose, including unwanted decor and unnecessary clutter.

- ☐ Surplus keychains and lanyards

- ☐ Unused pet accessories near the door

- ☐ Unused shoes that are kept in this space

☐ Organize

Redefine your entryway as both a charming welcome for guests and a practical launch pad for daily outings. This balance is key to maintaining both the area's appeal and its utility.

1. **Essential Items First:**
   - *Prioritize a space for everyday essentials (such as keys, wallets, and bags) using hooks or a small table. This ensures you can easily grab what you need on the way out.*

2. **Shoe Management:**
   - *Allocate a specific area for shoes using a rack or tray. Encourage household members to limit the shoes kept here to 1-2 pairs each to avoid overcrowding.*

Color coded sections of the home.

Follow-along discard checklist.

Learn what and how to organize with a clear step by step process.

Why Clutter Happens

No system of organization:

Without clear strategies or systems in place, items naturally find their way into random spots, leading to clutter.

Inconvenient storage solutions:

If an item's assigned location is hard to reach or use, it's unlikely to be returned there consistently.

Too much stuff:

Even with the best organization systems, storage solutions, and designated spots for every item, clutter can still occur if you simply have too much stuff. It will make any attempt at maintaining order too taxing and near impossible.

Items don't have 'homes:'

Every item should have a designated place. When you don't know exactly where something goes, you likely just place it somewhere random and leave it.

Underlying psychological factors:

Sometimes, clutter is a manifestation of deeper issues, such as habits formed from societal pressures or childhood experiences.

For instance, growing up with the notion of keeping things "just in case" or in an environment of scarce resources can lead to habitually holding onto items, whether needed or not. Addressing these roots with the help of a mental health professional can be crucial for lasting change.

Different Types of Clutter

Gretchen Rubin, author of the "*The Happiness Project*," has found there to be eight different types of clutter.

1. Nostalgic clutter

"Relics I clung to from my early life."

2. Conservation clutter

"Things that I've kept because they're useful - even though they're useless to me."

3. Bargain clutter

"Results from buying unnecessary things because they're on sale."

4. Freebie clutter

"Gifts, hand-me-downs, and giveaways that we didn't use."

5. Crutch clutter

"These things I used but knew I shouldn't," such as worn out or ill-fitting clothes.

6. Aspirational clutter

"Things that I owned but only aspired to use."

7. Outgrown clutter

"Things that I used to use but no longer need."

8. Buyers' remorse clutter

"Things that I kept rather than admit that I'd made a bad purchase."

Alternatively, Marie Kondo, a world-renowned tidying expert and author of "The Life-Changing Magic of Tidying Up," argues there are only 2 types of clutter:

When we really delve into the reasons for why we can't let something go, there are only two: an attachment to the past or a fear for the future.

The Decluttering Process

When Discarding

When deciding what to keep, you should ask yourself these three questions:

"Have I even used this item in the last year?"

"Does it still serve its intended purpose?"

"Am I actually excited to keep this item?"

Aim for a 'yes' on all counts for items that you choose to keep. If you find you're holding onto things that don't fit these criteria, it might be time to rethink why. Could it be because you think you should out of obligation?

For clarity, revisit the "Different Types of Clutter" outlined on Page 18. Evaluate whether the item in question falls into any of the described categories of clutter. Be honest with yourself during this decluttering process.

When Organizing

After completing the discard process, consider this while you reorganize:

"In what ways could my space be better organized to support my current lifestyle and my personal goals?"

In the process of organizing, prioritize grouping similar items, opting for a streamlined storage approach that's easy to manage, and ensuring that items you use frequently are within easy reach. Categorizing items by color, size, or usage can also help streamline your organization process.

If organization proves challenging, assess whether the space is appropriate for the items or if additional organizational tools (like shelves or bins) are needed to accommodate them effectively.

The Benefits
of Organization

Physical Health:

People in cleaner environments tend to be healthier than those in cluttered ones, with the benefits of being clutter-free often surpassing the health benefits of living in walkable neighborhoods.

Stress Levels & Productivity:

Reduced visual chaos lightens the brain's workload, leading to improved mental clarity, enhanced focus, and better relaxation. This supports effective coping strategies and boosts overall well-being.

A Few Quick Tips Before Getting Started:

- Use a timer for short, focused cleaning sessions if longer ones feel overwhelming.
- If you create a maybe pile while discarding, set a firm deadline to decide on those items.
- Take before and after pictures to visualize your progress.

Nutrition & Diet:

Tidy settings encourage healthier eating habits. For instance, people are twice as likely to choose an apple over a chocolate bar in a clean environment.

Relationships:

Enhance communication by reducing physical distractions, build confidence in hosting guests, and save time that would otherwise be spent managing clutter, fostering deeper connections with friends and family.

- Approach decluttering as if you're moving; keep only what you'd take with you.
- Remember, your kindness shouldn't lead to clutter; be mindful of what you keep.

Shaping Your Space to Shape Yourself

Understanding how your surroundings influence you is key to environmental psychology.

The principle of "person-environment fit" is a well-researched idea that highlights the importance of aligning your living spaces with your needs and goals.

For example, if you want:

- **To be healthy:** Rearrange your kitchen to make healthy food choices and cooking tools more accessible, encouraging better eating habits.

- **To encourage your kids' independence:** Place items your children use daily within their reach. This setup fosters their autonomy and instills a sense of responsibility.

- **To become a writer:** Create a clutter-free workspace in your home, complete with motivational decor and good lighting, free from distractions, to enhance your focus and bring your writing aspirations to life.

A dramatic reorganization of the home causes correspondingly dramatic changes in lifestyle and perspective.

It is life transforming.

Marie Kondo

The Spark

Your home organization journey ignites with an initial spark—a delicate flicker of motivation and determination.

It's in this beginning that the promise of a powerful transformation lies glowing, waiting to be fanned into a roaring flame.

Now let's be clear: success in this phase isn't about how long your decluttering sessions are or how many items you're getting rid of.

No, the real victory is in the act of showing up, in choosing commitment. Even if the first section seems intimidating, don't be discouraged.

Commit to just part of it. And if that still feels daunting? Do just a shelf or a drawer.

The key is to make showing up feel manageable as you navigate this initial phase. By focusing on action, no matter how small, you are progressing.

Every item sorted, every space organized, is a testament to your dedication. Your journey begins with this initial spark—a potent drive for change.

By consistently fueling this motivation with small steps and small successes, you will see that delicate flicker evolve into a roaring fire, driving your progress.

My main goal for this phase:

Living Room

The living room is often the heart of the home, a place where life's daily activities unfold. Despite being one of the most used rooms, it is frequently the messiest, serving as a magnet for clutter.

This section will guide you through decluttering and organizing to transform your living room into a haven of relaxation, comfort, and enjoyment.

Setting Your Intentions:

What part of the room immediately draws my attention, and why? Is it because I love that space, or because it is noticeably cluttered?

What activities take place here? Does the room's layout and organization support these functions effectively?

How do I want my living room to look and feel?

Furniture

Having set a vision for your living room, it's time to actualize it, starting with furniture.

Although you may not have a lot of furniture items, their size significantly impacts the room's openness, atmosphere, and flow. Thoughtful selection and arrangement of furniture pieces are key to transforming the space into your envisioned haven.

'Discard' doesn't always mean 'throw away.'

Consider selling or donating items that no longer fit your vision.

Regardless of how you choose to discard your items, be sure to follow through quickly to keep momentum in your living room transformation.

☐ Discard

DATE

When discarding, imagine you're about to move to a smaller home and need to review every possession for its value and necessity. This will make it easier to distinguish between what truly matters and what can be let go.

☐ Multiple or unused TVs

☐ Stained rugs

☐ Anything under your sofa cushions

☐ Lamps you don't use

☐ Unused furniture (couches, chairs, tables, etc.)

☐ Broken clocks

☐ Any piece of furniture you simply don't use or enjoy

Remember

When decluttering, ask yourself:
Have I used this in the last year? Does it still serve its intended purpose? Am I excited to keep it?

When organizing, ask yourself:
In what ways could my space be better organized to support my current lifestyle and my personal goals?

Living Room: Furniture

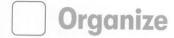 **Organize**

Start with a vision for your living room: think about the atmosphere you want and the feelings you're trying to create. Next, consider your furniture layout (you can sketch your plan on the following page) and be sure to take measurements beforehand to ensure furniture fits before any heavy lifting begins.

1. Optimize Furniture Layout:

- Visualize your ideal arrangement, considering traffic flow and natural focal points such as fireplaces or large windows.

2. Organize Furniture Storage:

- Empty out storage compartments in furniture like side tables, coffee tables, or storage ottomans. Discard what's not necessary, relocate what doesn't belong.

- Arrange items so frequently used ones are easily accessible, and store seldom-used items neatly out of sight.

Notes

Decor & Sentimental Items

Your living room's decor shapes its atmosphere, yet it's easy to fill this space with items out of habit or obligation.

Take a moment to look around. Are there decorations or keepsakes that no longer reflect your current taste? This step is about identifying what genuinely belongs in your living room and what's merely taking up space.

Letting go of physical clutter also declutters the mind and soul.

April Williams

Discard

You may be holding onto decor or items you're not fond of simply because they were gifts or you think they'll impress visitors. However, this approach doesn't help in crafting a space that truly resonates with you — the one who lives with it daily.

- ☐ Bulky or excessive decor and art pieces
- ☐ Dead plants or any unappealing plastic plants
- ☐ Unused lamps or lighting fixtures
- ☐ Old magazines and newspapers
- ☐ Wall art, signs, and posters you no longer love
- ☐ Candle holders, knick-knacks, and coasters that are outdated or broken
- ☐ Excess cushions or throws, including those that are worn out or mismatched
- ☐ Souvenirs with no sentimental value
- ☐ Broken, unused, or unattractive vases
- ☐ Unnecessary picture frames
- ☐ Decor pieces without personal significance or appeal
- ☐ Duplicate or unappealing photographs

☐ **Organize**

Photographs, with their deep sentimental value, present a unique challenge in this section. Choose images that reflect the desired mood and personal joy, with frames that align with your decor. For extensive collections, digital frames offer an elegant solution to display many memories without the clutter.

1. Choose The Decor Items You'd Like to Display:

- Select items that complement your living room's atmosphere.

2. Plan Placement of Decor Items:

- Decide on wall or surface placements, such as shelves or tables, ensuring you avoid cluttered arrangements.

3. Gather Necessary Tools and Materials:

- Prepare everything needed for displaying the decor items, including frames, hooks, etc.

4. Implement Your Plan

Notes

Electronics & Accessories

Living rooms often morph into entertainment hubs, cluttered with an assortment of devices and tangled cords.

This digital accumulation not only can overwhelm your space but also complicate your enjoyment of movies, music, and games in the space.

Streamline Your Subscriptions:

While organizing your physical electronics, take the opportunity to digitally declutter as well. Evaluate your streaming services and gaming subscriptions, canceling those you no longer use.

☐ Discard

Start by gathering all your electronics-related items—CDs, DVDs, video games, cases, cords, and remotes—into the center of the room. If the collection is large, tackle it in segments, such as CDs first, then DVDs, and so on.

Devices & Accessories

- ☐ Broken wires, devices, or consoles
- ☐ Wires for devices or consoles no longer owned
- ☐ Duplicate cords
- ☐ Unnecessary charging cords
- ☐ Remotes that are no longer needed or are broken
- ☐ Headphones or earbuds that are unused or not functioning properly
- ☐ Old devices (cameras, computers, phones) no longer in use
- ☐ Old tech accessories like phone cases no longer in use

Media

- ☐ CDs, records, tapes not listened to in the last 6-12 months that have no sentimental value
- ☐ DVDs not re-watched in the last 6-12 months that have no sentimental value
- ☐ Video games finished and won't replay
- ☐ Video games not played in years
- ☐ In-progress video games with no interest in finishing
- ☐ CD/DVD/video game cases with missing discs
- ☐ Discs that are scratched or too damaged to use

Living Room: Electronics & Accessories

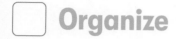 **Organize**

Not only is cord and device clutter visually - and therefore mentally - overwhelming, but it also makes things more difficult for you when you actually need to use it.

1. Group Electronics by Use:

- *Sort all devices, accessories, and media by their function. Group gaming consoles, audio equipment, and viewing devices together to streamline usage and access.*

2. Optimize Media Storage:

- *Choose a storage solution that fits your collection size and living room layout.*

- *Small collections: Consider entertainment center drawers, shelves, or zip-up storage binders.*

- *Large collections: Media storage cabinets or shelves dedicated to your media offer an organized and accessible solution.*

- *Organization method: Arrange CDs, DVDs, and video games alphabetically, by genre, case color, console type, or artist to find what you need quickly.*

3. Cord Management:

- *Go through all your cords and decide which you need accessible and which cords can be stored away.*

- *For cords you need to have accessible, consider cord management boxes and cable clips to reduce visual clutter.*

- *For cords stored away, try zip ties or color-coded Velcro strips to bundle like cords together, reducing clutter and facilitating easy identification for when you need to use them.*

4. Create a Tech Accessory Station:

- Designate a specific area in your living room for charging and storing tech accessories.

- Ideal locations include side tables with storage drawers or a designated shelf.

- Consider adding a wireless charging pad inside a drawer or on the tabletop to keep devices charged without visible cords.

5. Review Your Organization Plan:

- Once you've designated spots for electronics, managed cords, and decided on media storage, put everything in its place. Ensure that each item's location supports its use and enhances the room's functionality.

Notes

Bookshelves

Books are beacons of knowledge, creativity, inspiration, and entertainment. Bookshelves, however, are common sources of clutter.

It's time to declutter and reimagine these spaces as stylish, functional areas that reflect your personal tastes and enhance the living room's atmosphere.

Buying books and reading books are two separate hobbies.

And you don't have to read every book you bought; if you haven't even touched it since buying it, or you've tried to read it but just couldn't get into it, there's no shame in getting rid of it.

☐ Discard

As you sift through your book collection, challenge yourself to differentiate between sentimental value and practicality. It's about finding balance—keeping books that inspire, entertain, and serve you, while letting go of those that no longer add value to your life or space.

☐ Books you haven't touched in over a year and likely won't read

☐ Damaged or incomplete books

☐ Outdated textbooks or reference materials

☐ Duplicate copies

☐ Decor items that no longer match your aesthetic

☐ Unloved or broken decorative pieces and photo frames

Living Room: Bookshelves

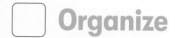 **Organize**

With a clearer bookshelf, it's time to think creatively about organization and display. This isn't just about arranging books; it's about designing a space that tells your story, showcases your interests, and brings joy every time you glance over.

---

1. Categorize Your Books:

- *Choose a method that appeals to you—be it by genre, color, or your personal reading journey.*

---

2. Incorporate Decor:

- *Select meaningful decor items that enhance the vibe you're aiming for. Balance is key; avoid overcrowding.*

---

3. Arrange Thoughtfully:

- *Place heavier items at the bottom and lighter, decorative items up top. Consider leaving space for both books and personal mementos to coexist beautifully.*

---

4. Implement and Adjust:

- *Set everything up according to your plan. Step back, assess, and adjust as needed to achieve the look and feel you desire.*

Notes

Games

Board games and puzzles offer timeless entertainment, creating cherished memories with friends and family. However, lost pieces, damaged boxes, and visual clutter from open storage can dampen the fun.

Owning less is better than organizing more.

Joshua Becker

☐ Discard

DATE

Letting go of board games and puzzles can evoke nostalgia, yet it's essential for maintaining a clutter-free space. Reflect on the last time each game was played and its condition. Discarding games that are no longer used or are missing pieces creates room for those you truly enjoy and use.

☐ Games with missing vital pieces

☐ Damaged games beyond playable condition

☐ Games untouched in the last 6-12 months

☐ Unused or incomplete games

☐ Outgrown children's games

Living Room: Games

☐ Organize

Effective storage of games and puzzles not only preserves their condition but also enhances your living space's aesthetics. The goal here is to make them playable, accessible yet unobtrusive.

1. Categorize Your Collection:

- *Sort games and puzzles by type or theme, such as board games, card games, and jigsaw puzzles. This categorization helps everyone find what they're looking for more quickly and encourages tidy habits.*

2. Dedicated Game Zone:

- *If space allows, designate a specific area or shelving unit in your home as a 'game zone'. This centralizes all game-related items, making them more accessible during game nights and helping maintain order.*

3. Optimize Storage:

- *Choose an area away from heat and moisture.*
- *Consider using protective sleeves for cards and zip-top bags or clear storage to keep puzzle pieces and game parts together. This not only helps prevent loss of pieces but also extends the life of your games and puzzles.*

4. Regular Maintenance:

- *Schedule regular clean-outs to reevaluate what you own. Dispose of or donate games that are no longer of interest, and repair or replace games with missing or damaged pieces.*

Notes

Milestone One Complete!

(1) ◯ ◯ ◯ ◯ ◯ ◯ ◯ ◯

You've finished decluttering and organizing your living room!

Revisiting Your Plan

Re-read the initial plan you wrote out on page 10. What hasn't been working for you and how can you address those pieces?

If you've missed any goals you've set for yourself, think about why that happened and how you can adjust your plan to account for similar situations going forward.

Alternatively, if things have been going well, pinpoint what's worked and how to sustain that momentum.

 Milestones are a space for you to celebrate your progress & revisit your foundation. There are 9 milestones spaced throughout this journey.

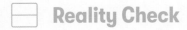

The Claim

"I'm just not built to be a clean or organized person."

The Reality

The drive towards cleanliness and organization is not just a personal preference but a deep-seated part of your psychology and biology, crucial for mental health and overall well-being.

You're Wired for Order

Your brain is naturally inclined towards order, loving patterns and predictability. This isn't just about liking things neat; it's about survival. From an evolutionary perspective, knowing your environment meant staying safe.

So, when you crave order, it's your brain doing what it does best—keeping you in tune with your surroundings.

This understanding can shift how you view your ability to organize, proving you're more than capable.

You Experience Mental Health Benefits When Your Space Is In Order

A tidy space isn't just pleasing to the eye; it's a boon for your brain. Organized environments can significantly boost your mood, sharpen your focus, and reduce stress.

These psychological rewards are your brain's way of thanking you for keeping things in order. It's clear evidence that being in a clutter-free state isn't just beneficial —it's preferred.

Your Brain is Created to Learn New Habits

Feeling like decluttering and organizing is out of your league? Here's some good news: your brain is built to adapt and change, thanks to neuroplasticity. Neuroplasticity is the brain's ability to reorganize itself by forming new neural connections throughout life.

This means you can develop new habits and preferences, including those for keeping your space neat and tidy. So, even if it feels like tidiness doesn't come naturally now, it can become a part of who you are with practice and patience.

Whenever you find yourself questioning your capability for cleanliness and organization, remember, your brain is on your side. Its inherent pull towards order and its ability to adapt and form new habits are powerful tools at your disposal.

Embrace your innate capabilities and watch how they transform not just your space, but your sense of self.

Kitchen

The kitchen is the culinary heart of the home, a place where meals are prepared, and often where families gather. As one of the most essential and frequently used areas, it can also become cluttered and disorganized, with countertops and cabinets overflowing with gadgets, utensils, and ingredients.

This section will guide you through decluttering and organizing to transform your kitchen into a space of efficiency, health, and culinary inspiration.

Setting Your Intentions:

Which part of my kitchen do I most often think about changing or improving? What specifically about this area stands out?

Reflect on your kitchen's primary roles—cooking, eating, entertaining, and supporting your health goals. Does its current organization enhance these functions, or hinder them?

How do I envision my ideal kitchen? What look and feel do I want to achieve?

Counter Space

Revitalizing your kitchen starts with maximizing counter space, the cornerstone of kitchen aesthetics and functionality.

Clear counters not only enhance the room's visual appeal but also streamline your cooking and preparation process.

Swap out the traditional knife block for a magnetic strip or in-drawer tray.

Knife blocks, while common, can consume valuable counter space, dull knives, and harbor bacteria.

A magnetic strip or drawer organizer saves space, keeps knives sharper, and promotes a cleaner kitchen environment.

☐ Discard

Kitchen counters often become a catch-all for various items, from seldom-used appliances to random non-kitchen objects. A clutter-free counter isn't just visually pleasing; it's essential for hygiene and efficiency in your food prep area.

☐ Unliked or damaged decor pieces cluttering the counter

☐ Excess or duplicate containers and packages

☐ Non-kitchen items that have found their way to the counter

☐ Expired or unused food products

☐ Any item that disrupts the counter's functionality or appearance

Remember

When decluttering, ask yourself:
Have I used this in the last year? Does it still serve its intended purpose? Am I excited to keep it?

When organizing, ask yourself:
In what ways could my space be better organized to support my current lifestyle and my personal goals?

☐ **Organize**

With the clutter gone, envision a counter space that complements your kitchen's purpose and your personal style. Consider the practicality of each item's placement, focusing on maintaining a balance between accessibility and aesthetic appeal. It's about creating a space that supports your culinary activities while being inviting and clean.

1. Reassess Decor:

- *Evaluate and minimize counter decor. Prioritize functional beauty that doesn't compromise space or risk damage from kitchen activities.*

⌄

2. Stow Infrequently Used Items:

- *Identify and relocate rarely used appliances and gadgets to free up counter space for essential daily activities.*

⌄

3. Rethink Spice Storage:

- *Move spices from the counter to a more protected, yet accessible, location to avoid clutter and contamination from cooking.*

⌄

4. Implement Your Plan:

- *Put your organization strategy into action, ensuring each item on your counter serves a purpose and contributes to the overall flow and functionality of your kitchen.*

Notes

Cookware & Dishes

Dive into the heart of your kitchen's functionality by sorting through cookware, bakeware, and dishes.

These essentials, when well-organized, not only streamline your cooking and dining experience but also infuse your kitchen with an air of readiness and calm.

A little polish goes a long way.

A versatile cleaner like Bar Keepers Friend can transform your kitchenware from dull to dazzling.

Discard

Gather all of your cookware and dishes into one central pile. This is your opportunity to carefully evaluate each item. One by one, determine what truly serves a purpose in your kitchen and what constitutes unnecessary clutter.

This process is not just about making space—it's about rediscovering and optimizing the essentials that make your kitchen functional and welcoming.

- [ ] Plates and bowls that exceed your daily needs, are rarely used, or are not in good condition

- [ ] Drinkware, including glasses, mugs, and water bottles, that exceeds your needs, such as duplicate sets or items that are rarely used

- [ ] Cookware and bakeware that are rarely or never used, including items like frying pans, saucepans, baking sheets, and muffin tins.

- [ ] Damaged dishes and cookware, including chipped, cracked, or warped items

- [ ] Pots, pans, and lids that don't have their matching counterparts

- [ ] Tupperware that doesn't have a matching lid, or any excess lids that don't have corresponding containers

- [ ] Fine china or special occasion dishes that don't align with your lifestyle

- [ ] Items with duplicates, favoring the ones in better condition

☐ Organize

With a curated collection of kitchen essentials, it's time to organize. Thoughtful placement not only streamlines meal prep but also turns your kitchen into a visually appealing space that reflects your personal style.

1. Define Zones:

- *Establish specific areas for cooking, prep, and storage. Position your tools close to where you use them most, like placing pots and pans near the stove and baking supplies near the oven. Keep related items together for intuitive use.*

⌄

2. Maximize Your Storage:

- *Most built-in kitchen cabinets have adjustable shelves. Use this to your advantage by customizing the shelf heights to easily accommodate large pots and tall dishes as needed.*

- *Utilize deep kitchen drawers for storing bulky items or creating a dedicated space for children's dining utensils that is easily accessible to them.*

- *Use stackable cookware sets or nesting bowls to maximize storage efficiency.*

- *Try specialized organizers like: lid organizers, plate racks, and adjustable cookware holders. These tools help keep items secure and maintain order within your cabinets.*

3. Focus on Accessibility:

- *Store everyday dishes and the cookware you use regularly in an easy-to-reach cabinet or shelf.*

- *Organize pots, pans, and lids by size and function. Place heavier items on lower shelves or in bottom cabinets to make retrieval easier and safer.*

4. Open Shelving:

- *Display your most frequently used and beautiful pieces on open shelves for easy access and aesthetic appeal.*

5. Seasonal Swap:

- *Rotate dishes and cookware based on seasonal use, keeping only the essentials within reach.*

Notes

Gadgets & Appliances

This section focuses on honing your arsenal of kitchen tools, ensuring each item genuinely enhances your cooking and prep experience without overwhelming your countertops.

Clutter is nothing more than postponed decisions.

Barbara Hemphill

☐ Discard

DATE

As you assess your collection of kitchen gadgets and appliances, prioritize functionality and utility. Reflect on their utility and frequency of use. It's time to part ways with those that have outlived their usefulness, are in disrepair, or simply don't make the cut in your cooking and kitchen routine.

☐ Unused gadgets and appliances

☐ Items that duplicate the function of others

☐ Outdated or malfunctioning equipment

☐ Appliances that are more hassle than help

☐ **Organize**

With a curated collection of kitchen gadgets and appliances, the next step is strategic placement. Optimizing your kitchen's layout involves not just aesthetics but also practicality, ensuring your most-used tools are accessible while infrequently used items are neatly stored away.

1. Prioritize Placement:

- *Assess which appliances you reach for daily and make sure these are readily accessible. Less frequently used items can be stored to preserve counter space.*

2. Strategic Storage Solutions:

- *Utilize cabinets, shelves, and even innovative storage solutions like under-cabinet hooks for small appliances to minimize clutter.*

3. Group by Use:

- *Keep similar appliances together to streamline your cooking process, making preparation smoother and more intuitive.*

Notes

Cutlery & Utensils

Overflowing drawers in the kitchen often turn finding a simple utensil into a frustrating task. It's time to tackle the excess cutlery and utensils cluttering your space.

Simplifying your kitchen drawers not only makes cooking more pleasant but also restores order and functionality to your daily meal prep.

Consider the convenience of hanging your most-used cooking utensils.

This not only saves precious drawer space but also keeps your tools within easy reach.

☐ Discard

It's time to confront the clutter. Start by emptying your drawers and counters, placing every piece of cutlery and utensil in view. This visual inventory will help you decide what's essential and what's expendable.

☐ Unused kitchen utensils

☐ Gifted cookware & utensils that you don't like or use randomly acquired cookware & utensils

☐ Dull or low-quality knives

☐ Excess or mismatched cutlery

☐ Duplicate measuring cups and spoons

☐ Organize

With unnecessary items gone, it's time to tackle the organization of your cutlery and utensils. Whether you opt for drawer dividers, wall-mounted solutions, or inventive storage hacks, the goal is clear: a kitchen where every item has its place.

1. Determine Storage Solutions:

- Decide on the best storage options for your cutlery and utensils, whether that's in drawers, on walls, or using creative organizers.

2. Implement Drawer Dividers:

- Use dividers or trays in your drawers to categorize and separate your utensils and cutlery, making each item easily accessible.

3. Arrange and Adjust:

- Place your items using the chosen method. Don't hesitate to adjust the layout until it perfectly suits your daily needs and enhances your kitchen's functionality.

Notes

Fridge & Freezer

The fridge and freezer are crucial in minimizing food waste and enhancing the kitchen's functionality.

By organizing these spaces, you not only improve visibility but also make healthier choices more accessible.

Introduce an 'Eat First' section or bin in your fridge to prioritize consuming foods nearing expiration.

Make sure these items are obviously visible so they're less likely to be forgotten.

71

☐ Discard

DATE

Tackling the fridge and freezer requires a mindful approach. Assess each item's usability, focusing on freshness and necessity. Make sure you're checking expiration dates for all the items in your fridge while discarding.

☐ Excess or outdated fridge magnets

☐ Outdated reminders or cards on the fridge

☐ Freezer-burned items

☐ Expired food products

☐ Unconsumed leftovers

☐ Partially used containers

☐ Unused ice cube trays

☐ Old or unused condiments and sauces

☐ Organize

Envision a fridge and freezer where everything has its place, from dairy to meats to ready-to-eat meals. Consider rearranging standard layouts to place healthier options, like fruits and vegetables, at eye level or in the door, making them the first thing you see and reach for.

1. Clean the Fridge and Freezer:

- *Before organizing, ensure all shelves, bins, and surfaces are cleaned. This step not only maintains hygiene but also gives you a fresh start.*

⌄

2. Categorize Your Foods:

- *Group items by type for easy access, emphasizing the placement of healthier options for visibility and convenience.*

⌄

3. Adjust Shelves and Bins:

- *Rearrange the fridge and freezer to suit your organizational plan, making efficient use of space for visibility and accessibility.*

⌄

4. Label and Date:

- *Mark all containers with contents and dates to monitor freshness and manage consumption effectively.*

Notes

Pantry

Navigating a cluttered pantry can be a daily frustration, leading to overlooked items and unnecessary purchases.

A streamlined pantry not only simplifies finding ingredients but also helps minimize food waste and overspending.

Streamline with Bins and Baskets:

For a clutter-free pantry, remove small, individually-wrapped snacks from their bulky boxes and store them in designated bins or baskets.

This is ideal for microwaveable popcorn, snack bars, fruit snacks, and bagged nuts or crackers.

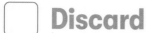

Discard

Embark on a pantry decluttering journey by gathering all items in one place. This will help you see exactly what you have, identify duplicates, and decide what's necessary.

- [ ] Expired or stale foods

- [ ] Foods you tried but didn't enjoy

- [ ] Unused condiments and sauces

- [ ] Old candies and snacks

- [ ] Foods in opened containers that weren't finished

- [ ] Items not fitting your current diet

- [ ] Unused party supplies

- [ ] Sprouted potatoes and onions

- [ ] Cookbooks and kitchen linens you don't use

☐ **Organize**

With a decluttered pantry, it's time to organize. A well-organized pantry not only looks appealing but also makes cooking more enjoyable and efficient. By creating specific zones for different types of food, you'll always know what you have and what you need.

1. Categorization and Zoning:

- *Assign specific areas in your pantry for various food categories, like baking supplies, snacks, and grains. This organization makes items easy to find and put away.*

2. Maximize Visibility and Space:

- *Use shelf risers, baskets, and door-mounted organizers to expand storage space and improve visibility.*

3. Label for Clarity:

- *Consider labeling zones, shelves, or containers to keep your pantry organized and prevent items from being misplaced.*

Notes

Spices

Spice cabinets often accumulate duplicates and rarely used seasonings intended for one-off recipes.

This section focuses on decluttering unnecessary spices and implementing an effective storage solution, ensuring your culinary creations are always flavored to perfection.

The first step in crafting the life you want is to get rid of everything you don't.

Joshua Becker

☐ Discard

While spices don't spoil in a traditional sense, their flavor diminishes over time. Keep this general guideline in mind as you evaluate and discard: seasoning mixes should be discarded after 1-2 years, herbs and ground spices after 1-3 years, and whole spices can last up to 4 years.

You can also do a quick potency test by smelling or tasting a small amount; if there's a noticeable lack of aroma or flavor, it's time to let go.

☐ Spices beyond their prime potency

☐ Unused spices lingering in your cabinet

☐ Seasonings that didn't match your taste

☐ Humidity-affected, clumped spices

☐ One-time recipe spices you haven't revisited

☐ Consolidate duplicates into a single container

☐ **Organize**

Storing spices away from heat, light, and moisture can significantly extend their shelf life, ensuring that your flavors remain potent and your meals delicious. As you prepare to organize your spices, consider a storage solution that keeps your spices easily accessible while preserving their quality.

1. Select Your Storage Method:

- *Choose between spice racks, cabinets, drawers, or pull-out units based on your kitchen layout and cooking habits.*

2. Preparation:

- *Clean the storage area and spice containers, ensuring everything is spotless before organization.*

3. Organization:

- *Utilize tiered racks for clear visibility and easy access. Avoid round storage options to maximize space and functionality.*

4. Labeling and Final Touches:

- *Ensure spices are clearly labeled. Consider using a consistent label design and font size for ease of reading and aesthetic appeal.*

- *Arrange them in a way that best suits your culinary flow, whether alphabetically, by frequency of use, or another system that works for you.*

Notes

The Sink

The area around your sink is pivotal for kitchen functionality and cleanliness.

This section aims to optimize space in, around, and below your sink, enhancing your kitchen's efficiency and aesthetic appeal.

Try the "room reset rule"
for maintaining tidiness.

Before leaving any room, reset it to its original state.

☐ Discard

DATE

Focusing on the sink area involves not just tackling visible clutter but also addressing the hidden messes below. It's time to purge items that detract from the space's cleanliness and utility, from outdated cleaning tools to under-sink storage hazards.

☐ Worn-out sponges or dish scrubbing brushes

☐ Damaged dishwashing gloves

☐ Germy dish drying racks

☐ Old steel wool scourers

☐ Unused dish soaps or detergents

☐ Unnecessary items under the sink

☐ Items susceptible to humidity damage

☐ Excess packaging materials like trash bag boxes

☐ **Organize**

After discarding unnecessary items, it's a good opportunity to assess how to maintain the sink area's organization and hygiene effectively. Consider if there are any cleaning supplies you're missing or need to replace.

Also, think about investing in organization tools for under-sink storage to keep essentials within reach and maintain a clutter-free space.

---

1. Streamline Your Sink Area:

- *Think about what you really use daily around the sink. Keep only those items out to minimize clutter.*

---

2. Maximize Under-Sink Storage:

- *Install pull-out drawers or shelves for easy access to cleaning supplies and use door-mounted racks for smaller items. Consider a waterproof mat or tray at the bottom to protect from water damage due to leaks.*

---

3. Consider Creating a Cleaning Caddy:

- *Assemble a portable caddy with essential cleaning supplies. This ensures you're ready for quick clean-ups, keeping your cleaning supplies functional and maintaining the organization with little effort.*

Notes

Milestone Two Complete!

1 2 ○ ○ ○ ○ ○ ○ ○

You've finished decluttering and organizing your kitchen!

Recalibrating Your Habit

The key to making habits stick is to make it easy. Does the difficulty feel fitting now and are there any adjustments you'd like to make?

If you feel overwhelmed by the idea of organizing a whole section of your home, what can you do to make it more manageable?

Consider breaking down the tasks even further, tackling one drawer or shelf at a time.

 A secret gift for you: Our team likes rewarding people who are continually taking small steps. To claim yours, scan here or email us now at **secret+homeorggift@habitnest.com**

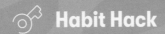

Habit Hack

Create a reward system to make dreaded chores feel manageable.

Why It Works:

The more tedious or daunting a task, the harder it is to muster the motivation to tackle it.

This lack of enthusiasm isn't a personal failing; it's rooted in human biology. Your brain is programmed to seek out rewarding activities, often leaving the less enticing tasks by the wayside.

To overcome this hurdle and address the tasks you're least looking forward to, establishing an effective reward system can provide the motivation you need.

There are four main types of reward systems you might consider:

1. Regenerative Rewards:

These rewards are all about rejuvenation and energy.

For Example: After completing a task, you might indulge in activities like a meditation session, a leisurely walk, a yoga break, a catch-up with a friend, or a favorite snack or drink. These activities allow you to relax and recharge, making them perfect incentives.

2. Concurrent Rewards:

These rewards are enjoyed while performing the task, making the process more enjoyable.

For Example: You might listen to music, podcasts, or even treat yourself to a special snack or drink to make the task more pleasant.

3. Cumulative Rewards:

Cumulative rewards build over time as you complete tasks.

For Example: You could add money to a gift card or a special savings account for each task completed, creating a fund for future treats or online shopping sprees.

2. Productive Rewards:

Productive rewards merge enjoyment with productivity enhancement.

For Example: Taking time to read a book that boosts your skills or listening to an educational podcast can be both rewarding and beneficial for your personal growth.

Experiment with these reward systems to discover what motivates you the most, and watch how setting meaningful rewards can dramatically alter your approach to even the most dreaded tasks.

Bedrooms

The bedroom is your personal sanctuary, a space for rest, relaxation, and rejuvenation. However, it can easily become cluttered and disorganized, affecting your peace of mind and quality of sleep.

This guide focuses on transforming your bedroom into an organized, tranquil haven that supports your well-being.

Start with your own bedroom, applying the principles laid out in this guide to create a space that truly reflects your needs and style.

You'll find instructions for children's bedrooms in the last section, tailored to accommodate their unique needs and activities.

For any additional bedrooms in your home, simply follow the same steps outlined here, adjusting as necessary to fit the room's specific purpose and the occupant's preferences.

Setting Your Intentions:

What area of the room first caught my attention, and why?
Is it because I love that space, or because it is noticeably cluttered?

What roles does your bedroom play in your daily life? Reflect on how these functions align with your needs for both rest and activity.

How do I envision my ideal bedroom? What look and feel do I want to achieve?

Furniture & Decor

Your bedroom is your personal comfort zone, where every bit of furniture and decor makes the space feel like yours.

It's a spot that should wrap you in comfort and reflect your unique style, giving you that perfect, peaceful feeling of being right at home.

Leverage versatile storage solutions like ottomans with storage compartments or decorative baskets to subtly manage clutter.

These can double as stylish decor elements while optimizing your space for calm and order.

Discard

It's time to reevaluate your bedroom's contents, focusing on furniture and decor that no longer serve your current lifestyle or aesthetic. If an item doesn't bring you joy or utility, it might be time to let it go, creating room for those that do.

- [ ] Mismatched or worn-out bedding and linens that detract from the room's comfort and appearance

- [ ] Decorative elements lacking personal significance or that clutter your space

- [ ] Furniture pieces that hinder movement or don't serve a current need, such as unused chairs or bulky dressers

- [ ] Out-of-place items that have migrated to your bedroom but belong elsewhere

- [ ] Lamps and lighting fixtures that are unused or malfunctioning

- [ ] Excess throw pillows or blankets that clutter the bed and are rarely used

- [ ] Unused or outdated electronics that contribute to visual and physical clutter

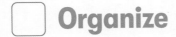 Organize

With the unnecessary items cleared out, it's time to create an environment that's both practical and deeply personal. Prioritize ease of use and the joy of living in a space that genuinely feels like yours, one that promotes rest and relaxation.

---

1. Visualize Your Ideal Bedroom Layout:

- *Consider the flow of the room. How do you move within the space? Place your furniture in a way that enhances movement and adds to the room's comfort.*

---

2. Choose Key Pieces of Furniture Wisely:

- *Identify the furniture that serves essential functions and contributes positively to the room's aesthetics. This might include your bed, a dresser, and perhaps a comfortable chair or a reading nook.*

---

3. Evaluate Lighting Options:

- *Proper lighting can transform the ambiance of a room. Consider adding dimmer switches, utilizing task lighting for reading areas, and placing decorative lamps to enhance the room's warmth and appeal.*

---

4. Declutter Surfaces:

- *Keep the tops of dressers, nightstands, and tables clear of unnecessary items. A minimalist approach can make the space feel more peaceful and organized.*

5. Organize and Display Decor Thoughtfully:

- *Arrange your decor in a way that showcases your personality while maintaining a cohesive look. Group items by theme, color, or significance, and avoid overcrowding shelves or surfaces.*

6. Implement Creative Storage Solutions for Small Items:

- *Use decorative baskets, trays, or boxes to organize smaller items like jewelry, glasses, or remote controls. This keeps them accessible but neatly contained. Utilize vertical space with shelves or hanging organizers to display decor or store items without crowding your bedroom.*

7. Finalize and Adjust:

- *Once all items are placed, take a step back to review the overall setup. Make any necessary adjustments to ensure everything feels balanced and aligned with your envisioned aesthetic.*

Notes

Nightstand

Your nightstand is a crucial element of your bedroom's functionality and aesthetic.

It's the last thing you interact with before sleep and the first thing you reach for upon waking. Keeping it organized and clutter-free can significantly impact your relaxation and sleep quality.

According to Feng Shui principles:

The height of your nightstand should not exceed your mattress's height to maintain energy harmony and accessibility.

☐ Discard

DATE

It's time to reassess the essentials and non-essentials on and within your nightstand. This process involves eliminating items that clutter this personal space, keeping only what contributes positively to your bedtime routine and morning start.

☐ Hygiene products that are empty or unused

☐ Writing tools and notepads that are unnecessary

☐ Empty or expired medication containers

☐ Broken or unnecessary alarm clocks

☐ Clutter including trash, on and within the nightstand

☐ Unused charging cables

☐ Damaged or unused eyeglasses

☐ Any other non-essential bedside items

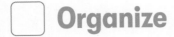 Organize

After clearing out the non-essentials, focus on curating a nightstand setup that's aligned with both your personal needs and the serene, restful energy ideal for a bedroom. Incorporate elements that aid relaxation, facilitate your bedtime and morning routines, and keep essential items organized and accessible.

1. Choose What Will Be on Your Nightstand:

Select items that directly contribute to your nighttime and morning routines, ensuring they enhance both functionality and comfort.

- **Essential Items:** *This includes items like an alarm clock, a lamp, perhaps a water glass or reading glasses. The key is to maintain accessibility while avoiding clutter.*

- **Personal Comfort Items:** *Add items that offer a personal touch and enhance comfort, like a favorite photograph or a scent diffuser with calming essential oils.*

- **Routine Support Items:** *Incorporate elements that aid your nightly routine and mental well-being, such as a gratitude notepad or a book, facilitating relaxation and sleep readiness.*

⌄

2. Organize Your Nightstand Drawers + Shelves:

Utilize drawers and shelves for items that you want within reach but do not need immediately at hand, maintaining organization and accessibility.

- **Accessible Items:** *Keep items that are part of your bedtime routine, such as lotions, sleeping masks, or extra charging cables organized and within reach but not cluttering the nightstand surface.*

- **Safety Items:** *Ensure emergency essentials, like a flashlight and necessary medications, are easily accessible yet securely stored.*

- **Organization Tips:** *Organize items by categorizing based on their use frequency. Employ drawer dividers or small containers for tidy storage, ensuring everything has its place.*

3. Manage Your Tech:

Strategically managing technology in your bedroom can significantly impact your sleep quality and overall relaxation. You can mix and match the following recommendations based on your needs.

a. **Surface Charging Station:** *Optionally, create a minimalistic charging station on the nightstand surface for essential devices, ensuring they're within reach but not cluttering the space.*

b. **Drawer/Shelf Charging Station:** *Alternatively, set up a charging station inside a drawer or shelf to keep devices out of sight, reducing blue light exposure before sleep.*

c. **Storing Devices Away:** *Consider storing devices away from the nightstand to minimize distractions before sleep, fostering a more restful environment.*

4. Review and Adjust:

• *After organizing, take a moment to assess your nightstand's setup. Ensure it aligns with your needs and promotes a tranquil, functional bedside area. Adjust as necessary to perfect your sleeping environment.*

Notes

Bedding & Linens

The abundance of bedding and linens in your home can quickly become overwhelming, especially when they start to accumulate without a clear organization strategy.

From overflowing linen closets to mismatched sets in our bedrooms, the clutter can detract from the comfort and aesthetics of your living spaces.

Consider using vacuum-sealed storage bags for out-of-season bedding to maximize closet space and protect your linens from dust and moisture.

☐ Discard

Begin by gathering all your bedding and linens. Aim to keep only those items that bring you comfort and match your current bedding needs. Remember, your bedroom is a personal space, meant to offer rest and relaxation.

☐ Bedding or linens that are worn out, torn, or stained beyond repair

☐ Duplicate items that exceed your actual needs

☐ Linens that no longer fit your bed size or your aesthetic preferences

☐ Any uncomfortable items that detract from a good night's sleep

Remember

When decluttering, ask yourself:
Have I used this in the last year?
Does it still serve its intended
purpose? Am I excited to keep it?

When organizing, ask yourself:
In what ways could my space
be better organized to support
my current lifestyle and my
personal goals?

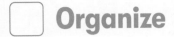 # Organize

Whether you have a dedicated linen closet or prefer to store linens in each respective room, the following tips are designed to bring order and accessibility to your bedding and linens. Remember, the goal is to create a system that works seamlessly for your lifestyle and space.

1. Fold Properly:

- *Begin by properly folding each item. Once folded, categorize your linens by type or by room, depending on your storage strategy.*

- *Note: If you struggle with folding sheets, try rolling sheets instead of folding them. Alternatively, online tutorials can be exceptionally helpful for mastering this skill.*

2. Store Strategically:

- *Decide on a storage location for each category of linens. Frequently used items should be easily accessible, while seasonal or spare sets can be stored higher up or in less accessible areas. Vacuum-sealed bags can be a great option for compact and protective storage of off-season bedding.*

3. Rotate Seasonally:

- *Make a habit of rotating your bedding according to the season. This not only helps with the wear and maintenance of your linens but also keeps your bedroom feeling fresh and appropriate for the temperature.*

4. Maintain Linen Freshness:

- Change your bed linens every one to two weeks to ensure cleanliness and reduce allergens. For a quick refresh and to minimize wrinkles, lightly spritz sheets with water and smooth them out after making the bed. This keeps your bedding inviting and comfortable.

Notes

Children's Bedrooms

Navigating the clutter in children's bedrooms can be a daunting task, with the space often transforming into a storage area for toys, clothes, and memories.

It's crucial to approach decluttering and organizing with strategies that respect both the sentimental value of items and the practical needs of a growing child.

Use a timer to make decluttering a game.

Even 5-10 minutes can motivate both you and your child to tackle the clutter in a fun way.

☐ Discard

DATE

Tackling clutter in children's bedrooms is not just about space; it's about making room for growth and change. The discard process might look different here, as it involves balancing the sentimental value of items with the practical needs of your child's current age and interests.

Evaluate what serves your child's present needs and consider a strategic approach for items still in good condition but no longer in use. Storing such items for future family growth or passing them on to friends or family can offer a practical and meaningful solution.

☐ Outgrown or unused clothing and shoes

☐ Toys that no longer capture your child's interest

☐ Broken or incomplete game sets and puzzles

☐ Books that are below your child's reading level or interest

☐ Any decor that doesn't fit the current theme or interest of your child

☐ Old school work and art that aren't chosen for keepsakes

☐ Unused or outgrown furniture pieces

☐ **Organize**

After decluttering, it's time to organize the room in a way that reflects your child's personality and supports their daily activities. From playtime to study time, every item should have its place, making it easier for your child to maintain a tidy room. If your child is old enough, be sure to include them in this process.

1. Categorize Toys and Books:

- Group toys and books by type or theme, making it easy for your child to find and put away their belongings. Use clear bins, shelves, or toy organizers to keep similar items together.

- Consider labeling bins with pictures or words, depending on your child's reading level, to foster independence in maintaining order.

2. Functional Furniture Placement:

- Arrange furniture to maximize play space and accessibility.

- Consider multifunctional pieces like storage benches or beds with built-in drawers for extra storage. Be sure all furniture is securely anchored, and storage solutions are at a height your child can safely access.

3. Create a Study Area:

- If your child is of school age, set up a dedicated study area with necessary supplies within reach.

- This can be a small desk or a corner of the room with organized storage for schoolwork and art supplies.

4. Implement the One In, One Out Rule:

- Teach your child the value of space and organization by applying the "One In, One Out" rule for toys and clothes - where for every new toy, book, or piece of clothing that is brought into the child's collection, one existing item must be removed.

- This encourages making thoughtful decisions about new items and helps prevent clutter from accumulating.

5. Personalize with Decor:

- Allow your child to choose some decor elements, giving them a sense of ownership and pride in their space. This can include wall art, a favorite bedding set, or a display shelf for their creations or collectibles.

Notes

Additional Bedrooms

As you extend your decluttering and organizing efforts to any additional bedrooms in your home, use the structured approach that you've already applied in your own bedroom.

Additional bedrooms often transition into storage spaces, accumulating belongings that are out of sight and, consequently, out of mind. Challenge yourself to evaluate whether these items truly serve a function or bring joy. If not, it may be time to let them go.

Use the space below to plan your space's purpose and include any notes that will help you evaluate and discard, as well as organize those rooms.

Check-in

Milestone Three Complete!

(1) (2) (3) ( ) ( ) ( ) ( ) ( ) ( )

You've finished decluttering and organizing your bedroom!

The Joy Factor

The more you enjoy your decluttering and organizing routines, the more likely you'll want to do them.

To seamlessly integrate this home organization journey into your life, reflect on how you can make it more enjoyable below.

Things to consider: Listening to your favorite playlist or podcast, involving family or friends, rewarding yourself after hitting a new milestone, etc.

The Ember

The Ember symbolizes both the stability you've attained and the potential that lies ahead.

Your steadfast determination has brought you to this phase. Now, the aim is to continue this momentum and take what you've learned into other areas of your home.

Maybe you've gotten better at letting clutter go, or maybe you've actualized your goal of doing a little every day to make it feel more manageable.

Now is your time to experiment.

Every adjustment, every tweak in your home organization journey to make it just a bit easier or enjoyable doesn't just maintain your momentum— it intensifies it.

And as the momentum builds, your home becomes more and more of a place you love, and ultimately a space and tool to support you and your goals.

Keep in mind: not every day will carry the spark of the start. If you ever find yourself struggling to declutter or organize, don't take it as failure but rather as feedback on what to adjust.

As you nurture and refine your home, remember: Every ember, when tended with care, holds the promise of a powerful blaze.

My main goal for this phase:

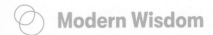
There is such thing as a "healthy mess"

A "healthy mess" navigates the fine line between clutter and an overly curated living space.

While excessive clutter can lead to stress, anxiety, and reduced productivity, an environment held to standards of perfection can be equally taxing.

The presence of a healthy mess can actually reflect a lived-in, vibrant home where life's moments unfold naturally.

This idea is not about embracing overwhelming clutter but about allowing your home to feel comfortable and genuinely reflective of your life.

Define What a Healthy Mess Is For Your Home:

The definition of what a "healthy mess" looks like is subjective and can vary greatly from one person to another.

Whether you're living solo or with roommates or family, reaching an understanding of what constitutes a "healthy mess" in your home can create a space that feels welcoming and comfortable for everyone and significantly reduce the potential for any resentment.

Reflect on your personal definition of a "healthy mess" or engage in a group discussion to align household expectations, using the following questions as a guide:

1. How do you define a "healthy mess"? What does that look like in different areas of your home?

2. What are the guidelines for maintaining a "healthy mess," and how are responsibilities shared?

3. Life changes, and so might your idea of a "healthy mess." How often will you revisit this to make sure you're hitting your goals?

Note: This check-in is also a great opportunity to acknowledge the effort being put into maintaining your home.

Clothing + Accessories

Clothing and accessories are extensions of your personality and a form of self-expression. Yet, closets and drawers often become cluttered with items no longer worn or needed, complicating the process of choosing outfits that reflect your current taste and lifestyle.

Statistics show that *the average person wears only 20% of the items in their wardrobe the vast majority (80%) of the time.*

This guide will help you declutter and organize your wardrobe, ensuring that your clothing and accessories serve you and your style well.

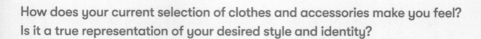

Setting Your Intentions:

How does your current selection of clothes and accessories make you feel? Is it a true representation of your desired style and identity?

Evaluate the current state of organization within your wardrobe. What specific organizational changes would most improve your daily routine?

How can you organize your wardrobe to enhance its visual appeal and make the clothing you want to wear more accessible?

Hanging Clothes

Starting with your hanging clothes is a strategic move to address a significant portion of your wardrobe and potentially free up closet space for better storage solutions.

This segment focuses on optimizing the organization of clothes hanging in your closet, ensuring every piece is something you love, fits well, and is ready to wear.

Add a second closet rod to maximize your closet's storage capacity.

☐ Discard

Decluttering your closet can be a daunting task, especially when faced with the thought, "I might wear this someday."

Evaluate each hanging item with a critical eye. Consider its fit, comfort, frequency of use, and whether it aligns with your current style and lifestyle needs or if you're keeping it for hypothetical scenarios that never seem to come. This process is about curating a wardrobe that genuinely serves you.

☐ Stained items that are beyond cleaning

☐ Damaged clothes that are irreparable

☐ Items you haven't worn in over a year

☐ Ill-fitting clothing

☐ Clothing that is to uncomfortable to wear

☐ Outfits unsuitable for your climate

☐ Professional attire no longer needed

☐ Outdated fashion unlikely to be worn again

☐ Special occasion attire with no future use

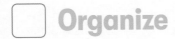 Organize

Post-declutter, organizing your hanging clothes by categories such as color, size, season, or function can streamline your daily routine, making outfit selection easier and more enjoyable. Consider the layout of your closet and how you can arrange clothes for ease of access, visibility, and care.

1. Define Your Organization Criteria:

- *Before rehanging your clothes, decide on the criteria that make the most sense for you. This could be by occasion (work, casual, formal), season (spring/summer, fall/winter), color, or type (tops, bottoms, dresses, outerwear). This step ensures you can find what you need quickly, matching your lifestyle and preferences.*

2. Implement Smart Storage Solutions:

- *To maximize closet space and maintain organization, consider adding slim, non-slip hangers, multi-tiered hangers for pants or scarves, and hanging shelves for lighter items. These tools can help keep your clothes in good condition and make the most of available space.*

3. Arrange Clothes with Accessibility in Mind:

- *Hang frequently worn items at eye level and within easy reach, while seasonal or special occasion wear can be stored higher up or in less accessible parts of the closet. This prioritizes ease of access for your daily routine.*

4. Leave Space Between Hangers:

- Avoid overcrowding by leaving a little space between hangers. This not only makes it easier to see and retrieve your clothes but also helps prevent wrinkling and damage.

5. Reassess and Rotate Seasonally:

- Every few months, take some time to reassess your closet organization. Rotate out seasonal clothing to keep your closet relevant to the current weather, and take the opportunity to donate or discard items that no longer fit your needs.

Notes

Dressers

Navigating a cluttered dresser each morning can start your day on a frustrating note. It's easy for dressers to become a catch-all for clothes we no longer wear or need, leading to drawers stuffed to the brim.

It's time to reclaim this essential storage space.

> Try drawer dividers to make the most of your space.

☐ Discard

DATE

Begin with an empty canvas by clearing out all dresser drawers. As you sift through each item, let go of those that fail to fit, comfort, or please you. Consider each piece's role in your wardrobe and life, choosing to keep only those that truly matter.

☐ Clothing that is beyond repair or stained

☐ Lonely socks and unmatched gloves

☐ Items that haven't been used in over a year

☐ Ill-fitting garments

☐ Extra buttons without a purpose

☐ Worn-out underwear and bras

☐ Pajamas that don't promise a good night's sleep

☐ Unused or ill-fitting swimsuits

☐ Tights with runs

☐ Organize

With a pared-down collection, organizing your dresser becomes a task of creative and mindful arrangement. Whether categorizing by color, season, or type, the goal is to fold and store items in a way that enhances both visibility and accessibility. Remember, the goal is to create a system that works for you and is easy to maintain.

1. Determine Your Organizing Strategy:

- *Decide on the best method for organizing your dresser drawers. You can organize by category (e.g., socks in one drawer, shirts in another), by color, by season, or even by frequency of use. Selecting a strategy that aligns with your lifestyle will make it easier to find what you need and keep everything in order.*

2. Master the Art of Folding:

- *Proper folding can significantly increase storage space and reduce wrinkling. Consider adopting the KonMari method of folding clothes into compact, upright packages. This technique not only saves space but also makes it easy to see all your items at a glance, preventing the need to rummage through stacks of clothes.*

3. Utilize Drawer Dividers:

- *To prevent items from getting jumbled, use drawer dividers or small boxes to create designated sections within each drawer. This is particularly useful for keeping smaller items like socks, underwear, and accessories organized and easily accessible.*

4. Implement the Vertical Storage Method:

- *Store folded items vertically, similar to files in a filing cabinet, to maximize space and visibility. This approach allows you to see every item without having to disturb the rest, making selection easier and keeping your drawers neater.*

5. Reassess and Adapt:

- *Once organized, take a step back to assess the setup. Make any necessary adjustments to ensure the system works for you in the long term. It should be easier now to make a habit of returning items to their designated spot after use or laundry.*

Notes

Shoes & Accessories

Sorting through shoes and accessories can quickly turn from a simple task into a walk down memory lane, filled with "maybes" and "what-ifs." It's easy to accumulate a collection of seldom-worn shoes and forgotten accessories.

This section aims to guide you through decluttering these items, making your space as functional and joyful as the pieces you choose to keep.

Incentivize your decluttering journey

Reward yourself upon completing a section's organization.

☐ Discard

As you go through your shoes and accessories, ask yourself if each item brings you joy or serves a purpose in your daily life. This mindset shift can help you let go of the unnecessary, making room for what truly matters.

Shoes

- ☐ Shoes that are worn out or damaged beyond repair
- ☐ Pairs you haven't worn in the last year
- ☐ Shoes that no longer fit comfortably
- ☐ Duplicate pairs that serve the same purpose
- ☐ Styles that don't match your current lifestyle or fashion sense

Accessories

- ☐ Jewelry that's broken or tarnished beyond cleaning
- ☐ Sunglasses with scratched lenses or frames
- ☐ Outdated prescription glasses
- ☐ Belts with worn-out holes or damaged buckles.
- ☐ Hats you never wear or that have lost their shape.
- ☐ Watches that no longer work or you don't wear
- ☐ Scarves that don't match your style or are damaged
- ☐ Ties you find unattractive or never wear
- ☐ Any accessory that doesn't make you feel confident when you wear it

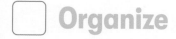 Organize

With the discarding phase behind you, it's time to bring order and accessibility to your remaining treasures. The goal is to create a system where every shoe has its place, and every accessory is easily within reach.

Shoes:

1. Evaluate Your Space:

- *Assess your current shoe storage solution and determine if it meets your needs. If not, consider alternative options like shoe racks, shelves, or an over-the-door organizer.*

2. Categorize Your Shoes:

- *Organize shoes by type (casual, sports, formal) or by frequency of use. This makes it easier to find what you're looking for and keeps your collection tidy.*

3. Implement Smart Storage:

- *Utilize space-saving strategies like storing shoes heel-to-toe or using clear shoe boxes for easy identification. For seldom-worn shoes, consider under-bed storage to free up more space in your closet.*

4. Maintain Accessibility:

- *Keep frequently worn shoes easily accessible, while seasonal or special occasion shoes can be stored away until needed.*

Accessories:

1. Sort by Category:

- *Separate your accessories into groups such as jewelry, belts, scarves, hats, and sunglasses. This simplifies the process of finding and choosing the right accessory for your outfit.*

2. Choose Appropriate Storage:

- *Select storage solutions that protect and display your accessories effectively. For jewelry, consider a jewelry box, drawer inserts, or wall-mounted organizers. For scarves and belts, use hangers or hooks for easy access.*

3. Maximize Vertical Space:

- *Utilize wall space or the back of closet doors for hanging accessories like hats, belts, and necklaces. This keeps them out of the way yet easily accessible.*

4. Dedicate Spaces:

- *Assign a specific spot for each type of accessory. This not only keeps your collection organized but also makes it easier to put things back in their place.*

Notes

Bags, Purses, and Luggage

Diving into the world of bags, purses, and luggage often reveals a common sight: bags stuffed inside other bags, a Russian doll scenario that seems practical until you're frantically searching for that one specific tote.

This section helps you untangle this nested mess so you can keep what's genuinely useful and part with the rest.

Out of clutter, find simplicity.

Albert Einstein

131

☐ Discard

DATE

You can accumulate a lot of clutter both inside your bags and with the bags themselves. This section focuses on addressing both types of clutter, streamlining your storage for better organization and ease of use.

Inside Bags

☐ Old receipts, tickets, and expired coupons

☐ Unused loyalty or membership cards

☐ Random bits of trash or forgotten items

☐ Old credit/debit cards or expired IDs

☐ Unnecessary duplicates of items (e.g., multiple lip balms or hand sanitizers)

☐ Broken or non-functional items (e.g., pens that don't work)

☐ Items that belong elsewhere but got stashed in a bag

Bags Themselves

☐ Duplicate bags that serve the same purpose

☐ Damaged or worn-out bags beyond repair

☐ Bags with broken zippers, straps, or closures

☐ Outdated bags that no longer match your style

☐ Bags that are uncomfortable to carry or use

☐ Unused promotional or freebie bags

☐ Bags you've outgrown or no longer have a use for

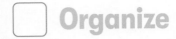

Organize

Efficient bag storage is key to keeping them in prime condition and easily accessible. Aim for a setup that respects their shape, protects them, and uses space wisely. Think about hanging smaller bags and using shelf dividers for larger ones, ensuring each bag is visible and ready for use. This approach not only saves space but also preserves your bags for longer use.

1. Visualize and Plan:

- *Determine how much space you have and how many bags need to be stored. Consider the types of bags and their sizes to plan your storage solution accordingly.*

2. Categorize Your Bags:

- *Separate your bags by type (e.g., purses, tote bags, luggage) and by frequency of use. This helps in deciding where to store them for easy access.*

3. Choose Your Storage Solutions:

- *For everyday bags, opt for hooks or a dedicated shelf near your entryway for grab-and-go convenience.*

- *Use clear boxes or shelf dividers for clutches and smaller bags to maintain shape and prevent them from getting lost among larger items.*

- *Consider hanging organizers or over-the-door hangers for frequently used bags, keeping them visible and accessible.*

- *For luggage and rarely used bags, utilize the top shelves of closets or under-bed storage containers to save space. You can also consider longer-term storage in a basement or garage if that's relevant to you.*

4. Implement Bag-In-Bag Storage:

- *For smaller bags, clutches, and seasonal items, store them inside larger bags to maximize space. This method also helps maintain their shape and protect them from dust.*

5. Maintain Accessibility:

- *Arrange your bags in a way that keeps your most-used items at arm's reach while storing seasonal or rarely used bags in less accessible spots.*

6. Label if Necessary:

- *If you're using boxes or bins, label them by category or season for easy identification. This step is especially useful for luggage and seasonal bags stored out of sight.*

Notes

Children's + Additional Clothing Closets

As you transition to organizing your children's clothes and accessories, leverage the strategies you've successfully implemented with your own wardrobe.

Remember, the closets and storage for your children's items should reflect their current needs and sizes, and be easily accessible to them. Involving your children in this process, if applicable, can teach them valuable organizational skills and help them understand the importance of keeping their spaces tidy.

Consider also the additional closets in your home, such as a separate coat closet or areas where you store seasonal items. Decide whether you want to tackle these now or wait until it's time to change over your clothes for a new season. This decision might depend on how frequently the items are used and the available space.

Use the space below to plan your approach for your children's clothing and accessories, as well as any additional closets.

Accountability
Check-in

Milestone Four Complete!

① ② ③ ④ ○ ○ ○ ○ ○

You've finished **decluttering and organizing your clothing and accessories!**

Dealing With Off-Days

It's normal to have days where you aren't feeling motivated to continue with your organizing journey or are feeling off in general.

What type of person do you want to be when these days inevitably come?

How would you like to act and manage your organizing goals on those days?

Never discard anything without saying thank you and good-bye.

Marie Kondo

Marie Kondo is a world-renowned organizing consultant and author, best known for her KonMari method of decluttering, which emphasizes keeping only items that "spark joy."

Embracing her approach transforms decluttering from a mere cleanup into a meaningful opportunity to reconnect with your surroundings and cultivate gratitude.

Using Gratitude in Your Decluttering Journey

Begin each decluttering session with a moment of reflection on the abundance that surrounds you.

As you evaluate each item, take a moment to express gratitude for its service or the joy it has brought you.

This gesture, rooted in respect and recognition, changes the process of parting with belongings from a challenge into a celebration of their significance in your life, thereby easing the decision to let them go.

Embracing Minimalism as a Mindset

As your journey progresses, consider embracing a minimalist mindset.

Remember, minimalism isn't about living with the bare minimum but about surrounding yourself only with things that matter - those that elicit a "yes" when you ask Marie Kondo's pivotal question: "Does this item spark joy?"

Decluttering is more than just removing items; it's about creating space for new experiences, joy, and peace. This minimalist approach promotes a lifestyle of intentionality, where every possession serves a meaningful purpose.

Bathrooms

The bathroom plays a crucial role in your daily routines and is your space for self-care. However, due to its functional nature, it can easily become cluttered with products, towels, and toiletries, sometimes making it one of the most challenging spaces to keep organized.

Setting Your Intentions:

What is your main organization goal for this area?

Consider how your bathroom is used daily. Does the current layout, setup, and organization support that purpose?

How do you want your bathroom to look and feel?

Shower & Bath Products

The bathroom, a sanctuary for cleanliness, often falls victim to the paradox of clutter, especially from shower and bath products.

With a mix of almost-empty bottles and an array of products for each family member, the space meant for cleansing becomes a hotspot for mess.

On bath, makeup, and skincare products, find the "open jar" symbol on packaging, indicating shelf life after opening. Located near the bottom or back of the product, It typically includes a number followed by "M," such as "6M" or "12M," indicating the number of months the product remains effective. Discard items that have been opened longer than indicated.

☐ Discard

DATE _____

Evaluate each product not just by its scent or promise but by its role in your routine. Ask yourself: Are you holding onto items out of habit? How practical is this item? When did I last use it, and does it still hold its effectiveness?

☐ Expired or nearly empty shampoo and conditioner bottles

☐ Bars of soap or body wash that you no longer use or like

☐ Unused items cluttering the shower caddy

☐ Old or worn out loofahs, sponges, and body poufs

☐ Disposable razors that have dulled or are past their prime

☐ Specialty products bought for one-time use

☐ Products that cause skin irritation or allergic reactions

☐ Expired sunscreens and skincare products

Bathrooms: Shower & Bath Products

☐ Organize

After decluttering, reimagining your shower and bath product storage becomes an exercise in accessibility and intention. By strategically placing items you wish to use more often within easy reach, you encourage their use. Conversely, items rarely used or needed for specific occasions can be stored out of immediate sight. This deliberate organization not only simplifies your routine but also ensures that products are used before they expire, minimizing waste.

1. Prioritize Daily Use Products:

- *Allocate prime real estate in your shower or bathroom to products you use daily, ensuring they are the first you reach for. This might include your favorite shampoo, conditioner, and body wash.*

2. Reposition for Encouragement:

- *Place items you want to use more but often overlook (such as treatments or masks) in a prominent spot. This slight change can remind and motivate you to incorporate them into your routine.*

3. Store Seldom-Used Items Strategically:

- *Identify a storage area for less frequently used products, such as guest toiletries or seasonal items. These can be kept in a cabinet, on higher shelves, or in storage bins under the sink, keeping them accessible yet out of the way.*

4. Implement Clear Storage Solutions:

- *Use transparent containers or labels for easy identification of products, especially for items stored out of immediate sight. This helps in quickly finding what you need without disrupting the order.*

5. Maintain a Rotation System:

- *For products with shorter shelf lives or those you're experimenting with, create a rotation system. This ensures that all products get used and prevents any from lingering unused for too long.*

Notes

Skincare & Makeup Products

It's easy to accumulate a wide range of products, from the miracle-promising serums to the latest eyeshadow palette that you just had to have. Yet, often, these treasures end up forgotten, gathering dust.

If your bathroom counters or drawers resemble a cosmetic graveyard, this section is your guide to reclaiming your space.

For new products or those you're unsure about, keep a dedicated "testing tray" where you place these items for a trial period.

If you find yourself consistently bypassing them, it might be time to pass them on.

Discard

The first step in decluttering your skincare and makeup is to confront the reality of unused, expired, or unsuitable products. It's easy to hold onto items due to cost or sentimental reasons, but if they're not serving you, they're only adding to the clutter. Remember, it's okay to let go.

- [ ] Makeup past its expiry date or that has changed in smell, texture, or color

- [ ] Makeup brushes and applicators that are frayed or impossible to clean

- [ ] Skincare products that caused adverse reactions or simply don't suit your skin type

- [ ] Samples or promotional items that didn't impress you or you never opened

- [ ] Duplicates of items where one will suffice or that you rarely use

- [ ] Any product you haven't reached for in the last 6-12 months

- [ ] Containers that are nearly empty or products you've been "saving" but never use

- [ ] Broken or malfunctioning beauty tools (e.g., eyelash curlers, tweezers)

- [ ] Excess nail polish colors you don't wear or that have become thick and clumpy

- [ ] Any beauty items that no longer fit your lifestyle, aesthetic, or beauty routine

☐ **Organize**

With the clutter out of the way, it's time to thoughtfully organize your remaining skincare and makeup products. The goal is to create a system that makes your daily routine smoother, keeps your products in good condition, and ensures you use what you have before it expires.

Prioritize accessibility for frequently used items and consider creative storage solutions to keep less-used products orderly yet out of the way.

---

1. Select a Storage Solution:

- *Choose between options like rotating makeup carousels, tiered spice racks for cabinets, clear acrylic organizers, over-the-door pocket organizers, or drawer organizing inserts based on your space and preference.*

---

2. Categorize Products:

- *Organize items by type or frequency of use to make them easily accessible. Keep daily essentials within reach and special occasion items together but out of the way.*

---

3. Maintain Tool Hygiene:

- *Store makeup brushes and tools in a clean, dry place. Consider using brush holders or separate containers to prevent cross-contamination.*

4. Implement a Use-First Area:

- *Designate a specific area or container for products that you want to use up first. Consider including product samples in this area as well. This can help reduce waste and ensure you're getting the most out of your collection.*

5. Seasonal Rotation:

- *If your makeup and skincare routine changes with the seasons, consider a seasonal rotation system. Store off-season items in a less accessible but organized area, swapping them out as needed.*

Notes

Hair Care & Styling Tools

Managing hair care products and styling tools can quickly turn into clutter chaos, especially with items like bobby pins and hair ties that seemingly vanish when you need them most.

He who buys what he does not need, steals from himself.

Swedish Proverb

☐ Discard

DATE

Streamlining your hair care and styling tools starts with acknowledging the essentials. Often, it's easy to accumulate a surplus of items like bobby pins and hair bands, thinking they're all necessary. As you sift through each item, consider not only its practically but also realistically assess the maximum number you actually use.

☐ Overstretched hair bands and scrunchies

☐ Hair dryer attachments that have never been used

☐ Unused, broken, or malfunctioning hair and beard trimmers

☐ Broken bobby pins or hair ties that no longer serve their purpose

☐ Duplicate or broken hair styling tools that clutter your space

☐ Hair care products you've tried but don't use or like

☐ Duplicate or unused hair brushes and combs that contribute to clutter

☐ **Organize**

Embarking on the organization phase for your hair care and styling tools invites a unique opportunity to redefine your routines. As you plan your new organizational structure, consider how to bring the most ease and joy to your daily hair care activities.

1. Categorize Your Items:

- Group your hair care products and styling tools by type. This could mean separating styling products, tools, and hair accessories. Use drawer organizers, bins, or baskets to keep similar items together.

2. Styling Tool Storage:

- For hairdryers, straighteners, and curling irons, consider installing a cabinet caddy or using hooks on the inside of cabinet doors. This keeps tools off the counter and cords neatly managed.

3. Implement a Cord Management System:

- Keep cords from becoming tangled by using velcro strips or cord wraps. This not only keeps your space tidy but also prolongs the life of your styling tools.

4. Accessory Organization:

- Use small containers or magnetic strips for bobby pins and hair clips to prevent them from scattering. For hair bands and scrunchies, a dedicated hook or a small basket can keep them organized and in one place.

5. Product Visibility:

- *Arrange hair care products in a way that you can easily see and reach for what you use most often. Tiered shelves or spice racks can be excellent for maximizing space and visibility in cabinets.*

6. Evaluate and Adjust as Needed

Notes

Medicine Cabinet

Navigating the maze of medications, supplements, and health aids requires a methodical approach to decluttering and organizing.

In a world blessed with advancements in healthcare, it's essential to ensure they contribute positively to your wellbeing without becoming clutter.

Always consult the FDA's website
or your local pharmacy for safe
disposal methods of expired or unused
medications to protect both your health
and the environment.

Discard

Holding onto medications and supplements past their prime can do more harm than good. This is a chance to clear out what's outdated or no longer beneficial, ensuring that your medications, supplements and any other health aids are current and actually helpful to your wellbeing.

- [ ] Expired medications

- [ ] Outdated or unused creams and ointments

- [ ] Outdated or unused over-the-counter drugs & vitamins

- [ ] Supplements you don't or won't use anymore

- [ ] Medications no longer actively prescribed or needed

- [ ] Unfinished prescribed courses of steroids or antibiotics (do not save for later use)

- [ ] Health aids past their expiry or in poor condition, such as bandages, antiseptics, and first aid supplies

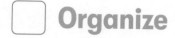 Organize

A streamlined medicine cabinet not only simplifies finding what you need but also ensures medications are stored safely and remain effective, whether you're managing daily medications or occasional remedies.

1. Implement a Sorting System:

- *Organize medications by type, purpose, or frequency of use, and consider various storage solutions like shelves, boxes, or drawers to accommodate different forms such as pills, creams, etc.*

2. Store Safely:

- *Ensure medications are kept in environments that don't compromise their efficacy—avoid places with extreme temperatures, moisture, or direct sunlight. Securely store away from children's reach.*

3. Optimize Daily Medication Management:

- *Utilizing pill organizers, from straightforward daily containers to advanced automated dispensers, can dramatically improve the ease and accuracy of managing your daily medication regimen.*

Notes

Towels & Toiletries

Whether it's a toothbrush that needs to be replaced or the towel collection that's seen better days, there are always items that linger longer than they should.

Decluttering towels and toiletries simplifies one of the most personal spaces in your home: the bathroom.

Stow away a stash of travel-sized
toiletries for guests.

☐ Discard

DATE

As you sift through towels and toiletries, challenge yourself to let go of the excess. Imagine opening your cabinets to find only items that you love and use, making each choice an act of self-care.

☐ Towels that are frayed, stained, or lack absorbency

☐ Rags no longer effective for cleaning

☐ Mismatched or faded linens that you avoid using

☐ Dental hygiene products past their prime, including toothbrushes older than 3-4 months

☐ Expired or disliked scented products, including air fresheners and candles

☐ Personal care tools like dull tweezers and nail clippers

☐ Hairbrushes and combs with missing bristles

☐ Unused or expired perfumes and colognes

☐ Travel-sized toiletries that are expired or unnecessary

☐ **Organize**

Adopt the mantra 'Everything in its place' to guide your organization of towels and toiletries. These items often end up scattered in various spots, leading to clutter and simply not knowing what you have.

Focus on consolidating and designating a single, logical home for each type of item to streamline your bathroom space.

1. Consolidate Categories:

- *Group all like items together. Keep all towels in one area and all toiletries in another to avoid spreading them across multiple locations.*

2. Designate Specific Homes:

- *Choose a primary spot for each category. For instance, all towels can be stored on a particular shelf or rack, while toiletries are kept in a designated drawer or cabinet.*

3. Prioritize Counter Space:

- *Maintain only essential items on the bathroom counter to avoid unnecessary clutter. Store surplus or infrequently used toiletries in accessible bins or cabinets.*

4. Utilize Organizers:

- *Employ drawer dividers, bins, and baskets to keep categories of toiletries neatly separated and easily accessible.*

5. Embrace Vertical Storage:

- *Use wall-mounted racks, over-the-toilet storage units, or over-the-door organizers to maximize space without spreading items out too much.*

6. Master Towel Folding or Rolling Techniques:

- *Learn and apply towel folding or rolling methods that best fit your storage space*

Notes

Children's Bathrooms

Similar to how you've organized your own bathroom items, now it's time to focus on creating a child-friendly environment that keeps their bath time fun and safe.

Sanitize bath toys weekly with a water and vinegar solution to eliminate bacteria and mold.

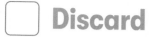

Discard

Children's bathrooms can quickly accumulate a variety of items, from bath toys to hygiene products. It's essential to regularly assess what's necessary, what's outgrown, and even what might pose a hygiene risk.

- [ ] Bath toys your child never uses or has outgrown
- [ ] Damaged, old, or moldy toys. Pay special attention to toys with hidden interior spaces where water can get trapped, like rubber duckies, squirt toys, and plastic figures with holes - these are prone to mold
- [ ] Empty or unused containers of soaps, shampoos, bath bubbles, or other bath additives
- [ ] Old toothbrushes (this should be replaced every 3-4 months, or immediately after illness)
- [ ] Expired skincare products
- [ ] Surplus hair accessories that are unused
- [ ] Unused bath products
- [ ] Old sponges or washcloths
- [ ] Excess bath mats or towels

☐ Organize

Adapting your child's bathroom for both functionality and fun is key. Consider storage solutions that not only keep items organized but also accessible to encourage your child's independence.

If they are old enough, include them in the process. This can be an excellent chance for them to learn about keeping their space tidy and making decisions about where things belong.

1. Sort and Store Bath Toys:

- Utilize mesh bags or dedicated bins for bath toys to allow for airflow and drying, reducing the risk of mold growth. Consider installing a toy hammock or suction cup baskets in the bathtub area for easy access and tidy storage.

2. Use Clear Containers for Small Items:

- Store hair accessories, small soaps, and other tiny items in clear, labeled containers. This makes it easier for your child to find what they need and encourages them to put things back in their place.

3. Designate Personal Hygiene Areas:

- Assign specific shelves, drawers, or sections of the medicine cabinet for your child's personal hygiene products. Label these areas if helpful to promote independence in their daily routines.

4. Implement Towel Hooks or Racks:

- *Install low towel hooks or racks that your child can easily reach. Encourage them to hang up their towel after each use to keep the bathroom tidy and allow towels to dry properly.*

Notes

Additional Bathrooms

As you move on to organize the extra bathrooms in your home, use the strategies you've applied to your own bathroom.

Additional bathrooms should not be a catch-alls for miscellaneous items and toiletries, concealing clutter from daily view.

Reflect on the specific uses of each bathroom to decide what stays and how to organize it. This could involve a mix of guest amenities, backup supplies, or specialized items for children.

Use the space below to plan for any additional bathrooms.

Milestone
Five
Complete!

(1) (2) (3) (4) (5) ( ) ( ) ( ) ( )

You've finished decluttering and organizing your bathroom!

A Moment to Celebrate

Incredible! You have now completed 5 major areas of your home and have shown serious commitment to get here.

Think back to where you were at the start of this home organization journey and consider where you are at now. Take this entire page to celebrate yourself and the progress you've made!

Enjoying your newfound habit? Help others find theirs. Scan this QR code to leave a review - it might be the nudge someone needs to begin their own life-changing journey.

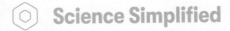

The Science Says

As little as one purchase can trigger a cycle of consumerism and clutter in your home

Coined in 1988, The Diderot Effect, named after French philosopher Denis Diderot, highlights how buying one new thing often leads to the desire for more.

This initial purchase can set off a chain reaction, where each new item seems to necessitate another, pulling you into a continuous loop of consumption.

In today's culture of consumerism, the message 'more is better' is everywhere, suggesting that happiness and fulfillment are tied to material possessions.

This mindset doesn't just hurt your wallet; it clutters your living space with items that soon lose their appeal, leaving you with a collection of things that don't serve a lasting purpose.

Finding its roots in the post-World War II era, consumerism, the notion that more stuff equals more happiness, has deeply influenced how society views success and identity, making it easy to equate personal worth with possessions.

Recognizing this pattern is the first step towards shifting your approach to buying. Opting out of the consumerist cycle means making more thoughtful choices about how you spend your money.

This reflection has lead many to try a new trend, called "New Consumerism," encouraging focusing on experiences over accumulating things. Investing in travel, hobbies, or cultural events not only enriches your life with meaningful experiences but also helps to combat the clutter that comes from unchecked buying.

By critically thinking about your buying motives and whether a purchase genuinely enhances your life, you can steer clear of the consumerism trap and make space for what truly enriches you and your home.

Misc. Indoors

You're making so much progress on your home organization journey! The goal of this section is to address any indoor spaces that you might have missed.

It may also be helpful for you to do a walkthrough of your home, and room by room think about any remaining odds and ends left to declutter and organize.

Setting Your Intentions:

Are there any spaces that feel disjointed or out of sync with the rest of your home?

Does the current layout and organization inside of your home support the purpose you have in mind? Are there underused areas that could be transformed with a clear purpose in mind?

Think about how your home is changing. What parts already match what you want, and what simple change(s) could make it even better?

Documents & Mail

Documents and mail can quickly become overwhelming clutter sources in any home.

With thousands of pieces of mail, including a significant amount of junk mail received over a lifetime, managing this deluge is essential for maintaining order and reducing stress.

Switch to digital whenever possible to reduce paper clutter.

Many services offer electronic statements and bills, which can help minimize the amount of physical mail you receive. Additionally, unsubscribe from unwanted catalogs and newsletters to keep junk mail at bay.

☐ Discard

As you sift through piles of papers, documents, and mail, focus on eliminating redundancy and irrelevance. Prioritize discarding outdated items, duplicates, or easily replaceable documents, and materials that no longer serve a practical purpose or hold sentimental value.

You should discard anything that is not sentimental and that does not fall into the following categories: currently in use, needed for a limited period of time, and must be kept indefinitely.

☐ Junk mail and irrelevant flyers

☐ Duplicated documents and outdated files

☐ Expired coupons and old receipts

☐ Magazines, newspapers, and clippings no longer of interest

☐ Excessive kid's school papers

☐ Unused instruction manuals and warranties

☐ Personal records that are no longer necessary

☐ **Organize**

Once you've decluttered, establishing a sustainable system for organizing the remaining documents is crucial. Aim for a setup that allows easy access to frequently used papers while securely storing those needed for the long term.

1. Categorize and File:

- *Divide remaining documents into categories based on their purpose or urgency. It may help you to use the categories you used while discarding: "currently in use", "needed for a limited period of time", and "must be kept indefinitely".*

- *Utilize filing cabinets, binders, or accordion files for efficient organization.*

2. Implement an Inbox System:

- *Designate a spot for incoming mail and documents requiring immediate attention. This could be a desktop tray or a wall-mounted organizer.*

- *When the task related to each paper is completed, remove it from your inbox and either shred it or file it away in the appropriate spot.*

- *If you prefer, you can get a second inbox tray so you can label one of them as urgent/time-sensitive and non-urgent.*

3. Create a Storage System for Sentimental Items:

- *For cherished items like children's artwork or significant letters, consider digital storage options to preserve them without physical clutter or create a specific space just for these sentimental items away from your to-dos.*

4. Routine Maintenance:

- *Regularly review and clear out your organized system to prevent backlog. Make it a habit to deal with new documents promptly.*

Notes

Home Office

Ever sit down to focus on your work, only to be overwhelmed by the clutter surrounding you? Surprisingly, the home office ranks as the second most cluttered area of the home, trailing only behind the garage.

It's time to transform this space from a source of stress to a productivity haven.

Keep a tray or folder for documents that need filing.

Set a regular reminder to file these documents to avoid pile-ups.

☐ Discard

DATE _____

If the mere thought of sitting down to work in your home office causes you stress, it's time for a change. Assess what genuinely serves your work needs versus what merely occupies space. It's not just about discarding; it's about making your workspace work for you.

☐ Non-functional or surplus office tools (pens, staplers, etc.)

☐ Electronics and cables no longer in use

☐ Stationery, mailing supplies, and business cards that are outdated or redundant

☐ Expired warranties or manuals for devices you no longer own

☐ Excess notebooks and notepads

☐ Outdated legal documents and old files with no legal or tax relevance

☐ Gifts or promotional items that don't add value to your workday

Misc. Indoors: Home Office

☐ Organize

Creating a visually appealing and organized home office is key to enhancing your productivity. Focus on simplicity and functionality in your workspace to minimize distractions and improve workflow. Good lighting and a touch of greenery can also boost your work environment's ambiance.

1. Designate Zones:

- *Create specific areas for different tasks—computing, filing, and brainstorming zones can help organize the flow of work.*

2. Optimize Desk Layout:

- *Arrange your desk with the items you use most within easy reach. This might mean having a good organizing tray for immediate essentials and a nearby drawer for secondary items.*

3. Invest in Adequate Storage:

- *If you find your desk is consistently cluttered with papers, consider adding a filing cabinet or additional shelving units dedicated to archiving.*

4. Digitize When Possible:

- *Embrace cloud storage solutions for document and photo storage to minimize the need for physical files.*

Notes

Entryway, Mudroom, & Foyer

A cluttered entrance can make coming home feel less like a relief and more like stepping into another chore.

Time to transform this space into a refreshing, organized welcome home.

Establish a
'Command Station'
in a central location
like the entryway.

This area can house a calendar,
to-do lists, and key reminders
to keep everyone aligned
and organized.

☐ Discard

Simplify your entryway to enhance its welcoming vibe. Remove items that don't belong or no longer serve a purpose, including unwanted decor and unnecessary clutter.

☐ Surplus keychains and lanyards

☐ Unused pet accessories near the door

☐ Unused shoes that are kept in this space

☐ Mysterious or obsolete keys

☐ Bulky furniture hindering the space's flow

☐ Decor that no longer matches your aesthetic or feels outdated

Remember

When decluttering, ask yourself:
Have I used this in the last year? Does it still serve its intended purpose? Am I excited to keep it?

When organizing, ask yourself:
In what ways could my space be better organized to support my current lifestyle and my personal goals?

☐ **Organize**

Redefine your entryway as both a charming welcome for guests and a practical launch pad for daily outings. This balance is key to maintaining both the area's appeal and its utility.

1. Essential Items First:

- *Prioritize a space for everyday essentials (such as keys, wallets, and bags) using hooks or a small table. This ensures you can easily grab what you need on the way out.*

2. Shoe Management:

- *Allocate a specific area for shoes using a rack or tray. Encourage household members to limit the shoes kept here to 1-2 pairs each to avoid overcrowding.*

3. Seasonal Swap:

- *Rotate items based on the season. Keep coats, scarves, and gloves accessible in winter, and replace them with sun hats and umbrellas in summer.*

4. Create a Mail Sorting Zone:

- *Avoid paper clutter by immediately sorting mail into categories like 'act now', 'file', or 'recycle'. A small basket or organizer can serve this purpose well.*

5. Child-Friendly Setup:

- For families, include lower hooks and shoe storage accessible to children, encouraging them to take responsibility for their belongings.

6. Visual Appeal:

- Keep the entryway inviting by incorporating elements of your home's decor style, such as a decorative rug, a vase of flowers, or art. This area should echo the warmth and style of your home's interior.

Notes

Hallways & Closets

Transform hallways and closets from mere passageways or storage catch-alls into organized, purposeful spaces.

A well-organized closet can serve more than just storage—it can simplify your life.

Under the influence of clutter, we may underestimate how much time we're giving to the less important stuff.

Zoë Kim

187

☐ Discard

Venturing into the hallways and closets can sometimes feel like opening a time capsule — items from the past that you've forgotten, mixed with the occasional 'I might need this someday.' Yet, these spaces are prime real estate in your home, meant to ease your daily routine, not complicate them.

☐ Outdated or unused photo frames and albums

☐ Long-stored items that have lost their utility or sentimental value

☐ Excess or damaged storage solutions

☐ Seasonal accessories like coats and scarves that haven't left the closet in years

☐ Spare linens and blankets that have been replaced or are no longer in rotation

☐ Miscellaneous items that somehow found their way into these spaces but belong elsewhere or need to be let go

☐ Organize

The key to an effective hallway and closet organization is clear definition and purpose. Determine what each closet is for—be it seasonal storage, linens, cleaning supplies, or guest necessities—and stick to it.

For hallways, aim for a welcoming and clutter-free passage.

1. **Assign Specific Functions to Each Closet or Area in Each Closet. For Example:**

   - *Seasonal Items:* include winter coats or summer beach gear. This keeps them out of the way when not in use but easily accessible when needed.
   - *Utility Items:* store cleaning supplies, vacuum cleaners, and other household tools.
   - *Guest Items:* guest linens, towels, and toiletries. This makes hosting easier and keeps guest items separate from your daily essentials.

   ⌄

2. **Maximize Vertical Space:**

   - Install shelves or hooks inside closets to utilize the full height of the space, perfect for storing lesser-used items on higher shelves and everyday items within easy reach.
   - Use door organizers for even more vertical storage.

   ⌄

3. **Label for Clarity:**

   - Use labels on shelves, bins, and baskets to clearly identify where items belong.

   ⌄

4. **Make a Schedule to Rotate Seasonal Items With The Seasons**

Notes

Laundry Room

Tackling the laundry room might not seem like a priority, given it's typically not overflowing with variety.

However, disorganization here can turn the already daunting task of laundry into an even bigger ordeal.

Your washing machine needs to be cleaned too. Every month or so, in an empty washing machine, run a hot cycle with 2 cups of white vinegar and 1/2 cup of baking soda, or use washing machine cleaner tablets. This helps remove residue and keeps your machine running smoothly.

☐ Discard

DATE

Stepping into your laundry room shouldn't feel like navigating through an obstacle course. As you declutter, focus on removing the unused, the unnecessary, and the obsolete.

☐ Detergents and fabric softeners that you've stopped using

☐ Empty or nearly empty containers of laundry supplies

☐ Specialty cleaning products that were never used

☐ Surplus or damaged laundry baskets and bins

☐ Unused or broken hangers cluttering the space

☐ Objects around your washer and dryer if they pose a fire hazard

☐ **Organize**

Designing an effective laundry workflow hinges on how well the space is organized. Whether you're working with a cozy nook or a spacious room, optimizing your laundry area can significantly reduce the time and effort spent on this household chore.

1. Maximize Your Space:

- *Utilize wall-mounted retractable drying racks and collapsible laundry baskets to save space. Install a retractable clothesline for air-drying and make use of over-the-door organizers for essential storage. This optimizes your laundry room's layout and functionality.*

2. Assign Baskets for Family Members:

- *Designate a laundry basket for each household member to simplify sorting and accountability.*

3. Assign Areas:

- *Set up specific zones within your laundry room for different tasks. Create a designated area for sorting dirty laundry, one for treating your garments, and another area with a flat surface for folding clean laundry to streamline the laundry process.*

4. Streamline Laundry Products:

- *Keep only the laundry products you use regularly. Try swapping out dryer sheets for wool balls to prevent residue on clothes and machines, and using white vinegar instead of fabric softener to avoid filmy residues.*

5. Label Everything:

- *Clearly label shelves, baskets, and storage areas to indicate where different items belong. This includes labeling areas for pre-treatment products, laundry detergents, and other supplies, making it easier for everyone to find what they need.*

6. Make It A Seamless Process:

- *Display a laundry symbols guide prominently for easy reference. Implement a laundry schedule to break down tasks throughout the week.*

- *Solve the mystery of missing socks by hanging a board or magnetic strip to hold single socks until their partners are found, clearing up space and keeping pairs together.*

Notes

Pet Items & Spaces

Pets are cherished members of the family, bringing joy, companionship, and unconditional love.

However, along with the wet kisses and happy tail wags, comes the challenge of managing their belongings - everything from toys scattered across the floor to grooming tools tucked in every corner.

> Camouflage pet gear by opting for storage solutions that align with your home's style, ensuring pet supplies enhance rather than detract from your decor.

☐ Discard

DATE
_____

Sifting through your pet's belongings might tug at your heartstrings, but it's essential to distinguish between what truly benefits your furry friend and what simply occupies valuable space.

☐ Expired or disliked pet treats

☐ Unused pet food bags

☐ Neglected pet toys

☐ Worn-out or excess pet toys

☐ Items from pets no longer with you

☐ Unused grooming tools (brushes, trimmers, etc.)

☐ Extra or unworn pet accessories (collars, leashes, etc.)

☐ Pet beds that are unused or in poor condition

☐ Unused, damaged pet cages or aquariums

☐ Organize

Dive into creating an orderly space for your pet's essentials, aiming to simplify both your lives. Give their belongings a proper home, reflecting the joy and companionship they bring into your home.

1. Establish Dedicated Zones:

- *Assign specific areas in your home for different pet needs. This can include feeding stations, grooming corners, and play areas. Clear zoning will simplify both your and your pet's daily routines.*

2. Optimize Food Storage:

- *Use airtight containers for pet food to maintain freshness, flavor, and nutritional value. Choose containers that fit well within your designated feeding zone, ensuring they're easily accessible yet out of the way.*

3. Streamline Leash and Accessory Storage:

- *Install hooks or a small shelf near your entryway for leashes, harnesses, and outdoor pet accessories. This keeps everything organized and ready for quick access during walks.*

4. Create a Toy Organizing System:

- *Dedicate a basket or bin for pet toys, preferably in or near their play area. Regularly rotate toys to keep your pet interested and engaged, storing away extras to avoid clutter.*

5. Grooming Supplies Station:

- Group all grooming tools and supplies in one portable caddy or drawer. This centralizes grooming essentials, making the process more organized and less time-consuming.

6. Implement a Cleaning Supply Kit:

- Assemble a cleaning kit specifically for pet messes, including urine cleaner, pet hair removers, and lint rollers. Store this kit in a central location to handle spills or accidents swiftly.

Notes

Hobby Items & Spaces

Think of your hobby space as a garden for your creativity. Just as a garden requires weeding to thrive, your space needs organizing to allow you to grow.

Organize your hobby supplies on a utility cart, making them conveniently mobile and ready to follow your muse.

☐ Discard

DATE

Embrace the hobbies that spark joy, and let go of the rest. Assess each item with a critical eye— if it no longer serves your current interests or projects, it's time to part ways.

☐ Supplies from hobbies you've moved on from

☐ Unused or expired arts & crafts materials

☐ Non-functional supplies

☐ Remnants and scraps from previous projects

☐ Projects you've lost interest in completing

☐ Hobby items, including musical instruments and related items gathering dust

☐ Any materials or tools that have been replaced by more efficient or updated versions

☐ **Organize**

Your hobby area shouldn't be a puzzle of misplaced items but a canvas for your imagination. Declutter and transform it into a space where every project feels like an adventure waiting to happen.

1. Segment Your Supplies:

- *Dedicate zones within your hobby area for different activities or projects. This could be as simple as having separate containers for painting, sewing, or electronic projects.*

2. Dedicate a Workspace:

- *If possible, allocate a specific area as your hobby zone. It doesn't have to be large; even a small desk or table can be enough.*

3. Embrace Vertical Storage:

- *Utilize wall space to hang tools, supplies, or even artworks-in-progress. Pegboards, magnetic strips, or simple hooks can transform unused wall areas into valuable storage spaces, keeping your work area clutter-free.*

4. Display Inspirational Items:

- *Reserve a spot in your hobby area for items that inspire you. Whether it's a mood board, your favorite artwork, or photos related to your hobby, having visual inspiration nearby can boost creativity.*

Home Gym & Exercise Equipment

Just as you fine-tune your exercise routine, it's time to fine-tune your fitness space. From weights to yoga mats, every item has its place so that you can hit your goals with ease.

People were created to be loved. Things were created to be used.

The reason why the world is in chaos is because things are being loved and people are being used.

John Green

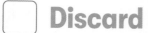 **Discard**

Your fitness journey evolves, and so should your space. Equipment that no longer aligns with your goals or is past its prime takes up valuable space. It's about crafting a space where you are excited to hit your fitness goals.

☐ Gear that has no use in your current fitness regimen

☐ Items worn beyond safe use

☐ Multiples you realistically never use

☐ Any tech or gadgets that have become obsolete

☐ Fitness DVDs and media you won't watch

☐ Exercise or yoga mats that are worn out/damaged

☐ Foam rollers that are damaged or not used

☐ **Organize**

Lean into wall storage to clear up your workout zone. With the right wall-mounted racks for your weights, bands, and mats, you'll keep clutter at bay and free up precious space for your fitness routine.

1. Streamline Storage Solutions:

- *Invest in smart storage that compliments your workout routine. Consider a sleek shelving unit for weights and an elegant stand for yoga mats and foam rollers.*

2. Zone Your Space:

- *Divide your area into workout zones—cardio, strength, stretching—to keep focused and flow seamlessly through your routine.*

3. Accessibility Is Key:

- *Ensure your most-used equipment is easily accessible. Less frequently used items can be stored out of immediate reach but still organized.*

4. Incorporate Inspiration:

- *Add elements that motivate you, whether it's motivational posters, a sound system for your workout playlist, or a small plant for a touch of nature.*

5. Maintenance Corner:

- *Dedicate a spot for cleaning supplies specifically for your equipment. Keeping your gear clean is as important as keeping it organized.*

Notes

Junk Drawers

The infamous junk drawer: every home has one, a catch-all for everything from old batteries to forgotten keys. But who says it has to be a source of chaos?

As you dive into your final indoor decluttering category, let's transform that drawer from a clutter catch-all to a neatly organized utility space.

Don't forget to reward yourself
for a job well done. You deserve it!

☐ Discard

Sifting through a junk drawer can often feel like an archaeological dig into your own home's history. Now's the time to empty it all out and carefully evaluate what you truly need. While some items may no longer serve a purpose and can be discarded, others may simply need to be rehomed to a spot where they're more useful.

☐ Old or unused phone cases that no longer fit your devices

☐ Instruction manuals for devices you no longer own or use

☐ Expired batteries and light bulbs that no longer serve their purpose

☐ Unnecessary electronics and devices that have seen better days

☐ Plastic membership or loyalty cards you never use

☐ Miscellaneous hardware items without a home or purpose

☐ Expired coupons or those unlikely to be used

☐ Party supplies that are past their prime or surplus to requirements

☐ Spare keys to unknown locks

☐ Glue or adhesive products that have lost their stickiness

☐ Loose change and neglected coin collections

☐ Rechargeable batteries that have lost their ability to charge effectively

☐ Organize

The goal isn't to eliminate the junk drawer but to refine it into a well-oiled utility drawer. It's about creating a space where essential tools and emergency items are at your fingertips, ensuring you're prepared for small tasks or unexpected repairs without the clutter.

1. Essential Utility Items:

- *Focus on including only those items that are genuinely useful in a pinch—think: flashlights, batteries, matches or lighters, tape, pens and pencils, scissors, glue, toothpicks, stain remover pens, eye glass repair kit, lint roller, zip ties, paper, envelopes, stamps, stapler, and screen wipes.*

2. Use Dividers:

- *Drawer dividers or small containers can help keep similar items grouped together, making them easier to find when needed.*

3. Designate a New Space for Common Clutter Items:

- *If you notice a collection of specific items, such as receipts or small knickknacks, that doesn't belong in the utility drawer, find or create a new dedicated space for these items where they can be easily accessed and organized.*

4. Label Sections if Needed:

- *Consider labeling sections within the drawer for even quicker access. Knowing exactly where to find your lint roller or eyeglass repair kit can save time and frustration.*

Notes

Milestone Six Complete!

① ② ③ ④ ⑤ ⑥ ○ ○ ○

You've finished decluttering and organizing all your indoor spaces!

Rekindling Your Spark

You have accomplished so much! As phenomenally as you're progressing, you may have noticed the initial spark you once had when starting may have dwindled a bit.

Take a moment to revisit the 'Why' you wrote out at the beginning of your journey on page 6. Does your why still resonate with you?

Write out any adjustments you'd like to make for it as you continue on with this journey.

The Blaze

The Blaze brings about better systems, big rewards, and lasting change.

From the first delicate spark of inspiration to the disciplined effort across every corner of your home, you've journeyed to the heart of The Blaze.

This is the phase where everything intensifies: the challenges, the rewards, and most importantly, the transformation.

It's in this radiant heat that you'll find yourself redefining what you thought was even possible. Your home looks totally different already, and now is the final push.

Every step you make to a more organized home, big or small, is a testament to your commitment to living a clutter-free life, and the new identity you are forging.

The rewards of this phase extend beyond momentary achievements, creating a home you love, that functions seamlessly for you, and acts as a foundation of support, not a project of perpetual labor.

But this blaze, as empowering as it is, comes with its own challenges.

Remember, while enjoying your successes, they stem from dedication and hard work. Don't become complacent; instead, use them as a foundation to propel you further.

As you continue to progress, your home organization systems solidify, rewards multiply, and you will emerge with an identity and a home that's been irrevocably changed for the better.

My main goal for this phase:

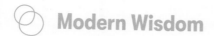

Challenging "What's The Point" and "What The Hell" Mindsets

The only limit to our realization of tomorrow will be our doubts of today.

Franklin D. Roosevelt

Decluttering isn't just about organizing your space; it can be a mental challenge that tests your perseverance.

Understanding and overcoming psychological hurdles can be the key to not just starting but also maintaining the motivation to declutter your home. Two common mental barriers stand out in this journey: the "What's the Point?" mindset and the "What the Hell" effect.

Common Mindset Challenges:

The "What's the Point?" Mindset

This thought pattern typically emerges amidst overwhelming clutter or discouragement from previous failed attempts. It's a mental trap that convinces you the effort isn't worth it because the task seems insurmountable.

This mindset can be paralyzing, preventing any action because the task seems too big or the benefits too small to matter.

If you catch yourself asking *"What's The Point"* it can be helpful to remind yourself of your "why" on Page 6 to help you reignite your purpose and drive.

The "What the Hell" Effect

This phenomenon occurs when a minor setback, like skipping a planned declutter session or finding an area cluttered again, spirals into abandoning the decluttering efforts entirely.

It's rooted in all-or-nothing thinking, where a perceived failure at a single task magnifies into a sense of total defeat that is beyond redemption. This mindset can derail decluttering efforts under the false belief that all progress has been undone.

If you catch yourself saying "What The Hell," take a moment to recognize setbacks are a normal part of the decluttering journey and do not erase the progress you've made. You can flip through the pages of this Transformation Journal for a visual reminder of your progress thus far.

 For additional support in overcoming mindset challenges, consider supplementing with tools like a motivation-boosting rewards system, detailed on Page 89.

Garage

The garage is often relegated to the role of a makeshift storage unit, a place where items you can't seem to part with, but derive no real use from, are stashed out of sight.

This "out of sight, out of mind" approach may seem like a temporary solution, but in reality, it only sweeps the problem of clutter under the rug, allowing it to grow unchecked.

As you embark on this journey, you're not just organizing a space; you're redefining its purpose. You will transform the garage from a forgotten storage corner into a functional, valued part of your home.

Setting Your Intentions:

What currently works in your garage and what doesn't? Is it cluttered with items you no longer use or need? Are tools and equipment hard to find?

What purpose do I want the garage to serve? Does it currently serve that purpose?

How do you envision your ideal garage space in terms of design and functionality?

Garage Instructions

1. Divide and Conquer:

Map out your current space into 3-5 distinct zones using the notes space on page 224.

This organization reduces overwhelm and allows you to focus on one area at a time; it's okay if it takes multiple days to fully sort through your garage.

2. Discard:

Refer to the categories listed on the next three pages as a guide for discarding items.

a. If your garage items are already sorted by the categories listed on the next three pages, work through each category systematically.

b. If your garage items are jumbled, use these categories to identify and decide on items to discard as you tackle each zone.

c. If your garage contains items that don't fit the categories listed on the next pages, such as cleaning supplies, home workout gear, extra kitchen gadgets, or hobby items, refer to the relevant category in this journal for discard guidance. Alternatively, use the notes space to list these additional categories.

3. Sort Items:

Form separate piles for items to keep, relocate to another area of your home, or discard.

As you sort, try to keep the 'keep' items organized by category within the garage itself. Promptly move any items you're relocating to their new spot, making sure that area is ready and organized to receive them.

4. Organize:

Follow the step-by-step guide on page 225 to design a new garage layout based on your current needs. Focus on grouping items by category to improve functionality.

 If uncertain, create a "maybe" pile for items, but be sure to set a deadline to decide their fate, ensuring they don't revert to clutter. This method allows for careful consideration without delaying your decluttering progress.

The Garage

This space often becomes a catch-all for a broad range of items, from tools to seasonal decor, necessitating a thoughtful approach.

Transforming your garage from a cluttered storage area into a functional, efficient space means you're not just reorganizing; you're reclaiming an essential part of your home.

Though it's just one part of this journey, don't underestimate the time and effort required.

Discard

DATE

Tools + Garden

☐ Old tires or auto parts not related to your current vehicle

☐ Spare tiles or flooring samples from previous projects

☐ Workbenches, shelves, or furniture that have lost their purpose

☐ Non-functional power tools or garden equipment

☐ Excess hardware like screws, nuts, and bolts without a specific project

☐ Unused gardening supplies, pots, and soil

Seasonal Items

☐ Outdated or irreparable items unfit for sale or donation

☐ Stored belongings that no longer serve a purpose in your life

☐ Malfunctioning holiday lights

☐ Excess or unused seasonal decorations

Continued on next page

Sports Gear

- [ ] Equipment for hobbies you no longer pursue

- [ ] Unused bikes, skateboards, and similar gear

- [ ] Damaged or excess fishing gear

- [ ] Beyond repair camping gear

- [ ] Unrepairable sports balls and inflatables

Electronics

- [ ] Outdated electronics

- [ ] Chargers and cables for devices you no longer own

- [ ] Broken electronics beyond repair

- [ ] Old batteries or electronic waste needing proper recycling

Kids Items

- [ ] Partially used outdoor play items like bubbles or chalk

- [ ] Sports equipment that your children have outgrown or no longer use

- [ ] Art supplies that have dried out or are otherwise unusable, such as markers, paints, and crayons

- [ ] Unused or broken electronic toys and gadgets

- [ ] School projects and artwork that aren't part of a curated keepsake collection

- [ ] Broken electronics beyond repair

- [ ] Baby gear and furniture that are no longer needed (cribs, high chairs, and baby swings)

Misc

☐ Irreparable items unfit for sale or donation

☐ Belongings that have outlived their usefulness

☐ Empty containers without a purpose

☐ Items that should be inside the house

☐ Items belonging to someone else that need returning

☐ Overlooked miscellaneous junk

☐ Unused or outdated cleaning solutions

☐ Items stored for others that have overstayed their welcome

Notes

More note space on page 227.

The Garage

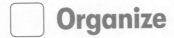

Organize

Envision your ideal garage use. Now is the time to plan. Designate different zones for various types of items, such as tools, gardening supplies, and sports equipment.

Use the notes space to outline which zones you'll create and the most functional storage solutions for each, considering their importance, frequency of use, and seasonality.

1. Establish Dedicated Zones:

- *Define and label your zones clearly. This organization will streamline maintenance and improve functionality.*

2. Evaluate Smart Storage Solutions:

- *Utilize shelving, hooks, and racks to maximize vertical space. Choose transparent bins for smaller items and label everything for easy identification. Prefer open shelving over cabinets for better access and visibility, minimizing hidden clutter.*

- ***For Tools and Workbench:*** *Organize tools on pegboards or magnetic strips, and keep small hardware in clear, divided containers.*

- ***For Sports and Outdoor Equipment:*** *Employ racks for bikes and balls, and hooks for bags and gear.*

- ***For Seasonal and Decor:*** *Use labeled bins for easy retrieval by holiday or season.*

3. Prioritize Accessibility:

- *Organize items by how frequently you use them. Keep daily essentials within easy reach, while seasonal items can be stored higher up or in less accessible spots.*

---

4. Enhance Safety:

- *Securely store heavy and hazardous materials to maintain a safe environment. Consider installing a carbon monoxide detector and an auto-stop feature on your garage door for added safety..*

---

5. Final Zone Check:

- *Review each zone to ensure it aligns with your current needs.*
  Be prepared to make adjustments as your lifestyle and hobbies change.

Notes   More note space on next page.

Notes

Milestone Seven Complete!

1 2 3 4 5 6 7 ○ ○

You've finished decluttering and organizing **your garage!**

The Progression Paradox

Have you found yourself being more lenient with what to keep or discard than you initially intended?

Instead of harboring guilt over these moments, consider whether you need to adjust your criteria to accommodate this leniency, or if you should recommit to the stricter guidelines you set for yourself at the start.

Things to consider: Is your current approach to decluttering accurately reflecting your organizational goals, or have the successes you've experienced led you to relax your standards more than you should? Are you giving yourself a "pass" because of the progress you've made, even if it means holding onto items that don't serve your space or your life as well as they should?

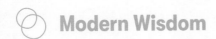

Organizing Around the World

From ancient practices that harmonize living spaces with the natural world to mindful decluttering rituals that ponder life's impermanence, cultures worldwide offer unique perspectives on organizing and decluttering.

Explore some intriguing global traditions that might inspire your organizing approach.

Danish Hygge: Coziness and Comfort

The Danish concept of Hygge emphasizes a warm, cozy, and comfortable home environment, promoting well-being and happiness.

To bring Hygge into your home, focus on incorporating soft lighting and candles to create a soothing atmosphere, adding plush textiles and comfortable furniture for physical warmth, and gathering spaces that encourage togetherness with loved ones.

Feng Shui: Harmony with Nature

Feng Shui, or "wind-water," is an ancient Chinese practice focused on spatial harmony to promote health and positive energy.

It encourages the use of natural elements—wood for growth, metal for logic and intelligence, water for wisdom and serenity—to create a balanced and tranquil home.

Central to Feng Shui is the art of arranging your space to optimize the flow of energy, or "qi."

For example clear paths to the front door for a welcoming vibe and avoiding blockages or positioning your bed in a way that allows you to have full sight of the door.

Swedish Death Cleaning: Mindfulness in Decluttering

Swedish Death Cleaning, or "döstädning," is a thoughtful decluttering process traditionally begun around the age of 50, aimed at minimizing the burden on loved ones after one's passing.

It's a proactive approach, undertaken while one is alive, to consider the future of possessions and the legacy left behind.

This practice involves a deep and reflective examination of each item's value, determining whether it should be kept, discarded, or gifted to someone now, rather than being sorted out later by family members.

It's a practice that underscores life's impermanence while fostering a sense of responsibility and care for those we will eventually leave behind.

Everything Outdoors

Just as you meticulously planned and organized each room inside your home, the exterior spaces deserve equal attention.

These spaces offer the first impression of your home and play a significant role in your everyday living experience, from gardening and relaxation to entertaining guests.

Begin by examining all your outdoor spaces —front yard, backyard, balconies, decks, and side areas. During this walkthrough, take a moment to evaluate the current condition of each area.

Setting Your Intentions:

What is your initial reaction to each outdoor area of your home?

What purpose do you want your outdoor space to serve? Does it currently serve that purpose?

How would your dream outdoor space look? What impression do you want it to give?

Outdoor Furniture & Cushions

Stepping into your outdoor area should feel like an escape —a place where comfort meets nature.

Whether it's a cozy corner on your balcony or an expansive garden, your outdoor furniture plays a key role in creating this sanctuary.

Protect your outdoor furniture and cushions with weather-resistant covers to extend their lifespan, minimize cleaning and maintenance, and help prevent mold buildup.

235

☐ Discard

DATE

As you approach your outdoor furniture and cushions, it's time to channel a sense of joy and practicality. Look at each piece closely and ask yourself if it truly enhances your outdoor experience. If it doesn't spark joy or serve a useful purpose, it may be time to let it go.

☐ Patio furniture and cushions that are damaged by wear, tear, or weather. Be sure to inspect underneath for any hidden issues like mold or structural weaknesses

☐ Furniture found to be ugly, unappealing, or uncomfortable

☐ Outdoor tables that are no longer wanted or needed

☐ Broken or unused porch swings

☐ Welcome mats that are damaged or unappealing

Remember

When decluttering, ask yourself:
Have I used this in the last year? Does it still serve its intended purpose? Am I excited to keep it?

When organizing, ask yourself:
In what ways could my space be better organized to support my current lifestyle and my personal goals?

☐ Organize

After decluttering, it's time to set the stage for your dream outdoor area. The objective is to arrange your outdoor furniture and accessories in a way that creates an oasis for relaxation and enjoyment.

1. Define the Purpose:

- *Determine the primary function of your outdoor space. Whether it's dining, lounging, or entertaining, align your furniture layout to facilitate these activities.*

2. Protective Storage:

- *Designate a storage solution for patio furniture cushions when not in use, such as a deck box or storage bench, to shield them from the elements and extend their life.*

3. Maximize Comfort:

- *Arrange seating to encourage conversation and relaxation. Incorporate additional comforts like outdoor rugs, pillows, and ambient lighting to elevate the space.*

4. Conduct Regular Safety Inspections:

- *Ensure the stability and safety of your deck and outdoor structures. Look for signs of wear, such as loose boards, unstable railings, or rot. Schedule annual inspections to catch any potential issues early.*

Notes

Grills & Fire Pits

Even these focal points of backyard entertainment can succumb to clutter, from worn-out tools to empty fuel containers. A tidy, well-arranged space invites more enjoyable, stress-free gatherings.

Use a storage bench or an outdoor cabinet near your grill or fire pit to neatly organize tools and essentials while providing protection from the elements.

☐ Discard

It's time to sift through your outdoor cooking equipment and fire-pit related gear. Pull all the tools and related equipment into a pile so you can see everything that you have.

☐ Worn or damaged grills and fire pits that are beyond repair

☐ Cleaning supplies and brushes that have seen better days

☐ Empty propane tanks or lighter fluid containers

☐ Depleted charcoal bags or wood chunks, leaving only what you'll use

☐ Worn out or damaged outdoor cooking utensils and tools

☐ Grill accessories that you haven't used in over a year

☐ Rusty or unsafe fire pit tools

☐ Any decorative items around the grill or fire pit area that are broken or no longer fit the aesthetic

☐ Protective covers for grills and fire pits that are torn or no longer effective

☐ Organize

Create a functional and inviting outdoor cooking and lounging area by thoughtfully organizing your grill and fire pit essentials. Focus on positioning these elements and their accessories for convenience, safety, and aesthetics.

1. Select Optimal Locations:

- *Determine the best spots for your grill and fire pit, considering wind direction, proximity to seating, and safety. Ensure they're placed on stable, non-flammable surfaces.*

2. Implement Tool Storage Solutions:

- *Hang metal tools like tongs and spatulas on wall-mounted hooks or magnetic strips, and store other accessories such as grill brushes and covers in a weather-resistant storage container. This keeps essentials within arm's reach and in good condition.*

- *Dedicate a small, easily accessible storage area for grill maintenance items like cleaning brushes, grill covers, and repair tools. Regular care extends the life of your grill and fire pit.*

3. Fuel Storage:

- *Safely store propane tanks, lighter fluid, charcoal, and wood in designated, well-ventilated areas away from direct heat sources. A locked cabinet or a sturdy outdoor box can prevent accidents and keep supplies dry.*

4. Accessorize for Efficiency and Safety:

- *Keep a fire extinguisher, grilling gloves, and long-handled tools nearby to handle high temperatures safely.*

∨

5. Seasonal Care:

- *If applicable, cover your grill and fire pit during off-season months or invest in durable covers to protect them from weather damage year-round.*

Notes

Pools, Floats, & Supplies

Dive right in to decluttering your pool area—it's time to make those sunny summer days even more enjoyable by transforming your poolside into a streamlined oasis where relaxation and fun are the only things on your agenda.

> # You can journey to the ends of the earth in search of success, but if you're lucky, you will discover happiness in your own backyard.

Russell Conwell

☐ Discard

Sifting through pool supplies might feel like wading through water, but it's essential for a splash-ready space. From outdated toys to unused chemicals, let's clear the way for hassle-free fun under the sun.

☐ Weather-worn or faded pool floats and toys.

☐ Pool covers that have seen better days, with tears or fading

☐ Surplus floaties and life vests, especially those that don't fit anyone anymore

☐ Chemicals past their prime, remembering safety first when disposing

☐ Abandoned kiddie pools, cracked or faded by the sun

☐ Organize

Just like a smooth swim, organizing your pool supplies should feel effortless and rewarding. It's time to create a streamlined system that makes every pool day a breeze, ensuring your supplies are protected and ready to go.

1. Designate Specific Storage Areas:

- *Choose a location like a garage, shed, or pool-house for storing pool supplies. Outdoor storage chests can also be a practical and aesthetic option.*

- *Use durable, clearly labeled containers to segregate toys, chemicals, and cleaning equipment, making sure everything has its designated spot.*

2. Store Floats & Toys in Reach:

- *Dedicate specific bins or mesh bags for floats and toys. This keeps them accessible, dry, and in good condition.*

3. Implement a Chemical Safety Zone:

- *Choose a secure, ventilated space for chemicals, away from direct sunlight and moisture. Use lockable cabinets if necessary for child and pet safety.*

4. Organize Maintenance Gear:

- *Hang cleaning supplies and pool maintenance tools on wall-mounted hooks or in a dedicated storage box to keep the area neat and tools in good condition.*

- *Designate an easily accessible area for pool covers, ensuring they're kept clean and ready for use to protect your pool when not in use.*

5. Seasonal Rotation:

* At the end of the season, assess your pool supplies. Store away off-season items and make a checklist of what needs replacing or repairing for the next pool season.

Notes

Lawn Ornaments & Decorations

Transform every corner of your outdoor area into a masterpiece where each lawn ornament and decoration is perfectly placed, with no clutter in sight.

Use app-controlled LED lighting to easily change your outdoor space's ambiance for seasonal flexibility, from festive holiday glows to vibrant summer hues.

☐ Discard

Embark on a garden declutter with an artist's eye—each piece should contribute to your outdoor masterpiece. Weed out the mismatched and worn, making room for decor that truly resonates with your aesthetic and joy.

☐ Faded or broken lawn ornaments that no longer sparkle

☐ Decorative lights that have lost their glow, year-round or seasonal

☐ Overlooked debris and dead foliage that dampen your garden's spirit

☐ Outdoor lighting fixtures that don't brighten your space as they should

☐ Past-season wreaths and signs that don't reflect your current style

☐ Flags and poles that have weathered beyond recognition

☐ Unused plant pots that clutter rather than cultivate

☐ Garden hoses that have sprung their last leak

☐ Organize

View your garden as a living gallery, where each piece contributes to the overall ambiance. It's about striking a balance between beauty and function, creating a space that invites you in and holds you in its charm.

1. Define Zones:

- *Clearly define areas in your garden for relaxation, entertainment, and visual interest. Use decorations to highlight these zones, creating seamless transitions between different uses of your outdoor space.*

2. Lighting for Mood:

- *Strategically place lighting to enhance the ambiance at night. Solar-powered lights offer an eco-friendly solution to highlight paths and features.*

3. Seasonal Rotation:

- *Keep your outdoor space fresh by rotating decorations according to the season. This also gives you a chance to maintain and repair any wear and tear.*

4. Storage Strategy:

- *Develop a systematic approach to storing off-season decorations to keep them in good condition for their next use. Consider vacuum-sealed bags for soft items like cushions and watertight bins for others.*

Outdoor Children's Toys

Dive into decluttering outdoor children's toys to create a tidy, safe play area. As birthdays and holidays pass, it's easy for new toys to overshadow old favorites, leading to a cluttered yard.

Never organize what you can discard.

Unknown

☐ Discard

DATE

Tackling the clutter of outdoor toys is a step towards reclaiming your backyard's tranquility and playfulness. Gather all toys in one spot and assess which ones still have a place in your child's heart and your outdoor space.

☐ Toys with wear or damage from outdoor elements

☐ Items with potential hazards like rusting metal or broken parts

☐ Outgrown bikes, scooters, and skateboards

☐ Toys that have lost their appeal to your child

☐ **Organize**

A well-organized outdoor toy storage solution not only protects toys from weather damage but also keeps your yard looking neat. Embrace a system that accommodates your child's current interests and the durability needs of outdoor playthings.

1. Weatherproof Storage:

- *Invest in durable, labeled weatherproof bins or outdoor storage chests to protect toys from sun and rain damage.*

⌄

2. Toy Rotation:

- *Apply the one-in-one-out rule to outdoor toys just as you might indoors, ensuring a manageable collection that fits your space and your child's interests.*

⌄

3. Accessibility:

- *Store toys in a way that makes them easily accessible for play and easy to put away. Consider the height and reach of your child when organizing.*

Notes

Vehicles

Vehicles often serve as an extension of your home, a place where you spend a considerable amount of time.

Just as cleanliness and organization are crucial in your living space, your car deserves the same level of attention for a clutter-free ride.

> **Install a dedicated, sealable trash container in your car to help keep things clean during your commutes.**

☐ Discard

Embark on a thorough cleanup of your vehicle by removing everything, including trash, items stashed in compartments, and anything beneath the seats. This decluttering drive ensures that only essential and meaningful items accompany your journeys.

☐ Stickers that are outdated or no longer reflective of your personal style. For easy removal, gently heat them with a hairdryer and peel off slowly

☐ Air fresheners that are old and scentless

☐ Unnecessary items in car door storage spots

☐ Misplaced items and clutter in cup holders

☐ Clutter in the trunk that lacks purpose

☐ Non-essential contents in the glove compartment

☐ Items tucked into the visor/mirror without function

☐ Outdated insurance cards, registrations, or maintenance

☐ **Organize**

Remember, a clutter-free car is a safer car. It minimizes distractions and makes necessary items easily accessible in emergencies.

1. Strategic Organizers:

- Utilize seat-back organizers for essentials, ensuring easy access without cluttering the space.

2. Essentials Kit:

- Maintain a compact box in the trunk, armrest, or glove compartment containing hand sanitizer, lotion, scissors, tape, pens, a sewing kit, stain remover, and necessary tools.

3. Document Management:

- Keep important car documents like registration, insurance, and maintenance records in a dedicated, easily accessible folder.

4. Seasonal Items:

- Designate a specific area for seasonal necessities such as ice scrapers, sunshades, or an umbrella, ensuring they're readily available when needed.

5. Organize Charging Cables:

- Dedicate a specific compartment or pouch for storing charging cables and electronic accessories.

6. Prepare for Emergencies:

- Assemble an emergency kit including water, non-perishable snacks, a first-aid kit, flashlight with extra batteries, blankets, jumper cables, road flares or reflective triangles, a multi-tool, a portable battery charger, maps and compass, a rain poncho, a whistle, and a seatbelt cutter with a window breaker tool.

- Store this kit in a compact, easily accessible location in your vehicle to ensure you're prepared for any situation on the road.

7. Implement Regular Clean-Outs:

- Make it a habit to remove trash and personal items after each car use to prevent accumulation.

Notes

Milestone Eight Complete!

1 2 3 4 5 6 7 8 ○

You've finished **decluttering and organizing your outdoor areas!**

Actualizing Aspirations

You have decluttered and organized every corner of your home, both inside and out. In doing so, you have proven to yourself you are a person who is clutter-free and organized. And now you get to reap the benefits of the new lifestyle you have designed.

When you began this journey, you described in detail on page 8 who you aspired to become. Flip back and reread what you wrote there now.

How has your identity changed since then?

Is there anything you still want to shift within yourself?

Science Simplified

The Science Says

Your brain is wired to seek immediate gratification, often leading you to buy or keep items for that instant satisfaction, even if it adds to clutter.

Akrasia, the Greek term for acting against one's better judgment, is a significant factor in the accumulation of home clutter.

This phenomenon was explored by philosophers such as Socrates and Aristotle. Today, this behavior aligns with what's known as hyperbolic discounting, a tendency to prefer smaller, immediate rewards over larger, later ones.

Hyperbolic discounting illustrates why you might opt for the short-term satisfaction of buying something new or keeping unnecessary items instead of the long-term benefit of a clutter-free space.

Recognizing this tendency can be crucial in addressing and overcoming the challenges of decluttering and maintaining your homes.

By setting small, manageable tasks, you can cater to your brain's craving for immediate gratification while progressively working towards the larger goal of an organized, clutter-free environment.

Going deeper into the science behind this — this method makes your dopamine release work for you, enhancing satisfaction with each small task completed, and capitalizes on the Goal Gradient Hypothesis which suggests that your motivation to complete tasks strengthens as you near your goals.

Setting smaller, achievable goals like you have in this Transformation Journal transforms the daunting end goal of decluttering your home into a series of motivating, attainable steps, making the journey towards a clutter-free environment both rewarding and manageable.

Keep that momentum going as you move forward into maintaining your new found home organization structure.

Maintenance Plan

After you've put in all this effort to declutter and organize your home, setting up a maintenance routine is key.

This section will outline a series of suggested tasks designed to keep your home clean and organized based on your new home organization system.

To ensure consistency and timeliness, tasks are categorized into daily, weekly, and monthly activities. Remember, these suggestions are a starting point—you should adjust them according to your needs, your living space, and your lifestyle.

It's also the perfect moment to discuss the maintenance plan with other household members or any hired help to ensure everyone is on the same page of who is responsible of what.

Life is dynamic, and your home's maintenance needs will evolve. Stay flexible and periodically review and tweak your routine to keep it effective and aligned with your changing circumstances.

Setting Your Intentions:

Identify the essential maintenance tasks that underpin your home's organization and cleanliness. What measures will you put in place to ensure these tasks are consistently completed?

Considering your daily schedule and lifestyle, what strategies can you use to make your maintenance routine both efficient and effective, minimizing effort while maximizing results?

What benchmarks will you set to measure the effectiveness of your maintenance routine, and how often will you reassess these benchmarks to ensure they still serve your home's needs?

Daily Checklist

Living Room

☐ Clear clutter hotspots

☐ Tidy up the couch + furniture

☐ Straighten up the shelves

Kitchen

☐ Empty and run dishwasher as necessary

☐ Wipe down countertops, surfaces, and high-touch appliances

☐ Wash out the sink, including any remaining dirty dishes

☐ Empty trash as needed

Bathroom

☐ Hang towels to dry

☐ Quick wipe down of sink and countertops

Bedroom

- [ ] Make your bed

- [ ] Clear clutter from dresser, desk, and nightstand

- [ ] Clear any items from the floor

Clothing + Accessories

- [ ] Put dirty laundry in basket

- [ ] Put away any clean laundry

- [ ] Put your clothes and accessories away after you remove them

Misc. Indoors

- [ ] Sort mail and papers into the inboxing system you created

- [ ] Clear any clutter from floor in hallways and entryways

Outdoors

- [ ] Water plants as needed

Weekly Checklist

Living Room

☐ Sweep, vacuum & mop floors

☐ Wipe down coffee table & surfaces

☐ Dust all surfaces

☐ Dust the bookshelf and books

☐ Clean floor under furniture

Kitchen

☐ Sweep, vacuum & mop floors

☐ Sort through food items in the fridge, tossing what's no longer fresh

☐ Clean inside the microwave. *Tip: to make it easier to clean grime, create some steam by heating a bowl of water for 5 minutes*

☐ Sanitize sponges. *Tip: you can do so by running it in the dishwasher, giving it a vinegar bath, or just putting it in boiling water for 5 minutes*

☐ Clean any remaining appliances

Bedroom

- [ ] Change sheets and pillowcases

- [ ] Vacuum and mop floor, don't forget to clean under the bed

- [ ] Switch out towels, including hand towels and wash cloths

- [ ] Dust surfaces

- [ ] Wipe down window sills

Clothing + Accessories

- [ ] Straighten out closet and dressers

Bathroom

- [ ] Sweep, vacuum & mop floors

- [ ] Empty trash cans

- [ ] Switch out towels, including hand towels and wash cloths

- [ ] Clean mirrors

- [ ] Wipe down shower, tub, sink, and handles

Maintenance Plan: Weekly Checklist

Misc. Indoors

☐ Sweep, vacuum, & mop floors of any hallways, entrances, and additional spaces

☐ Wipe down laundry machines, clean out any leftover lint

☐ Wash pet bowls and clean any pet bedding

Garage

☐ Clear clutter hotspots

☐ Sweep floors

Outdoors

☐ Clear clutter hotspots

☐ Wipe down and dust high-use surfaces like outdoor tables and furniture

Notes

Monthly Checklist

Each month, take a walkthrough of every room to evaluate whether clutter is creeping back or if your current systems are actually meeting your needs. Regular monthly reviews help ensure your home stays organized and functional.

Should you find the need to declutter and reorganize, you can always return to the relevant section of this Transformation Journal.

Living Room

☐ Dust baseboards & ceiling fans

☐ Vacuum furniture

☐ Wipe down light switches and doorknobs

Kitchen

- [ ] Take inventory of freezer items that need to be tossed, eaten soon, or restocked

- [ ] Wipe down fridge shelves & drawers

- [ ] Clean inside of oven or toaster oven if necessary

- [ ] Clean inside the dishwasher if necessary

- [ ] Spot clean tile-grout and backsplash

- [ ] Wash trash can

Bedroom

- [ ] Wash duvet covers, comforters, and other blankets

- [ ] Dust the ceiling fan

- [ ] Dust blinds and baseboards

Clothing + Accessories

- [ ] Put away out-of-season clothes, and bring out any stored clothing & accessories for the current season as needed

Maintenance Plan: Monthly Checklist

Bathroom

☐ Clean and organize cabinets and drawers

☐ Check & restock toiletries and cleaning supplies as needed

☐ Wash trash cans

Misc. Indoors

☐ Wash remaining trash cans

☐ Dust remaining ceiling fans

☐ Clean vents and air filters

Outdoors

☐ Sweep deck and balcony floors

☐ Wash outdoor cushions as needed

☐ Wipe down outdoor umbrellas as needed

☐ Clear away any dead weeds or leaves

☐ Trim and prune plants and needed

Garage

☐ Dust surfaces

Notes

Maintenance Reflection

Reflect on your maintenance plan in the space below.

Consider: Who will be responsible for each task? How will you ensure the plan is not just implemented, but sustained over time? What are the mechanisms for accountability and adaptability within your approach to keep your home clutter-free, clean, and organized?

Milestone Nine Complete!

(1) (2) (3) (4) (5) (6) (7) (8) (9 ✓)

You've finished decluttering, organizing, **and learning to maintain your home!**

Shaping a Resilient Identity

It's inevitable that your life will have different seasons, some drastically different than the one you're currently in.

Take this page to revisit your identity through a more long-term lens.

How can you expand your desired identity to be more resilient despite the different ways your life may change going forward?

Home Transformation

Organization
Journal
Complete! Volume 1

Celebrate your journey!

Every small step you've taken has led to this moment.
Share your success using #HabitNest

With small steps, you've made some big changes.

You began this journey ready for a change. Now, after decluttering and organizing every corner of your home, you can confidently say you've finally become clutter-free.

Both you and your home have transformed immensely since your first day.

Should you ever feel your habits wavering, always know that Habit Nest is there for you, welcoming you back, ready to rekindle your spark once more.

So, What's Next?

Use the space below to make a plan to continue your progress.

Consider which tools and resources you will use to maintain this plan.

Shop Habit Nest

Ready to set new habit goals? We're here for you.

This whole journey may have lit the fire in you to address other habits in your life. Whether you're eager to tackle more habits personally or inspire someone else, our range of habit-building products awaits to elevate your journey even further.

Get More

The Habit Nest App

Experience behavior change on the go with a beautifully designed mobile experience available on the App Store and Google Play Store. Claim your 7-day free trial today. Learn more at **habitnest.com/app**

The Phoenixes

Want your own VIP access pass to all things Habit Nest? Get your Phoenix digital collectible at **habitnest.com/vip**

Volume 1

Home Organization Transformation Journal

Finally become clutter-free.

ISBN 978-1-950045-26-6

9 781950 045266

90000>

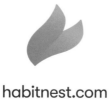

habitnest.com